Therapy To Go

by the same author

Therapy To Go
Gourmet Fast Food Handouts for Working with Child,
Adolescent and Family Clients
Clare Rosoman
ISBN 978 1 84310 643 2

of related interest

The Art of Helping Others
Being Around, Being There, Being Wise
Heather Smith and Mark Smith
ISBN 978 1 84310 638 8

The Expressive Arts Activity Book
A Resource for Professionals
Suzanne Darley and Wende Heath
Illustrated by Mark Darley
Foreword by Gene D. Cohen MD PhD
ISBN 978 1 84310 861 0

Art Therapy and Anger
Edited by Marian Liebmann
ISBN 978 84310 425 4

Working with Adults with Asperger Syndrome
A Practical Toolkit
Carol Hagland and Zillah Webb
ISBN 978 1 84905 036 4

Best Practice in Professional Supervision
A Guide for the Helping Professions
Allyson Davys and Liz Beddoe
ISBN 978 1 84310 995 2

An Integrative Approach to Therapy and Supervision
A Practical Guide for Counsellors and Psychotherapists
Mary Harris and Anne Brockbank
ISBN 9781843106364

Art Therapy and Creative Coping Techniques for Older Adults
Susan I. Buchalter
ISBN 978 1 84905 830 8

Helping Adolescents and Adults to Build Self-Esteem
A Photocopiable Resource Book
Second Edition
Deborah Plummer
ISBN 978 1 84310 185 7

Therapy To Go

Gourmet Fast Food Handouts for Working with Adult Clients

Clare Rosoman

Jessica Kingsley *Publishers*
London and Philadelphia

First published in 2008
by Jessica Kingsley Publishers
116 Pentonville Road
London N1 9JB, UK
and
400 Market Street, Suite 400
Philadelphia, PA 19106, USA

www.jkp.com

Library of Congress Cataloging in Publication Data

Rosoman, Clare.
  Therapy to go : gourmet fast food handouts for working with adult clients / Clare Rosoman.
     p. cm.
  ISBN 978-1-84310-642-5 (pb : alk. paper)
  1. Psychotherapy--Problems, exercises, etc. 2. Patient education. I. Title.
  RC480.5.R6675 2008
  616.8'4910654--dc22

                                        2008014822

British Library Cataloguing in Publication Data
A CIP catalogue record for this book is available from the British Library

ISBN 978 1 84310 642 5

Menu

Main Course

Dessert

APPETISERS

How to use this book

This book is designed to be a quick and easy 'fast food' resource for all kinds of therapists working on a professional level with adult clients. Whether you trained as a counsellor, psychologist, social worker, psychiatrist or psychotherapist, there are activities in this book that can help all therapists to work towards their therapeutic goals with their clients. This book provides fast 'take-away' activities that cover a wide variety of presenting problems. Each activity is presented in worksheet format and can be photocopied for therapists' use with their clients.

The worksheets intend to complement or expand upon the treatment plan that has already been determined by the client and the therapist. This book is not designed to be a treatment manual and the sheets are not designed to be used in any particular sequence. Rather, it aims to be a stimulus for ideas and creativity in therapy. It is intended that the therapist will pick and choose amongst the worksheets, selecting those activities that will help them to best meet the therapeutic goals.

It is assumed that the professionals using this book have a sound grounding in counselling and diagnostic skills. The book aims to offer a wealth of ideas for activities and techniques to use with clients, so reducing the preparation time for sessions. For therapists of all levels of experience, it offers suggestions for different, creative approaches to difficult client issues and can help avoid the need to develop therapy resources, which can be time-consuming.

To receive the most from this resource, it is helpful to peruse the worksheets to become familiar with them, then to select the activity or a range of activities that are likely to suit the client's presenting concerns. This means that the therapist can take a flexible approach to each session by having a variety of exercises available to use, and can therefore allow the client to determine the direction of discussion.

At the start of each section there is an explanation of each activity, including a description of how the sheet could be used in therapy; however, this serves as a guide for the therapist only.

Why worksheets?

Worksheets are a valuable therapeutic tool because they are visual, direct and structured. They vary the process of therapy and can provide a framework for the content of a therapy session. This book aims to compile a large amount of commonly needed therapy tools in order to save the therapist time and to provide immediate, 'fast food therapy tools' to be used with their clients.

For the client, worksheets are easy to read and are visually appealing. They are non-threatening because they contain limited amounts of information and they can be worked through to the client's self-determined level of comfort. They provide a sense of safety because the client can see the activity or questions before they commence an activity and can feel in control of how deeply they expose themselves.

Worksheets can guide the content and process of therapy by opening up discussion and exploring deeper issues that the client may feel happier writing down or thinking about first. The sheets in this book aim to provide a variety of ideas to help therapists to guide their client's discovery.

One of the values of worksheets is that they can be taken home by the client. This means that the information contained on the worksheets can be digested over time and taken out of the therapy room to be read and re-read, stuck up on the wall as a visual prompt, or can be shown to friends and family members. This may encourage the generalisation and inter-contextualisation of therapeutic progress. This is, after all, what therapy is all about: applying the therapeutic strategies to life outside of the therapy room.

Clinical issues

The worksheets and activities in this book aim to assist the therapist in:

- forming rapport with the client and hearing the client's story
- determining treatment goals and the client's motivation to change
- using specific techniques to explore the client's experiences
- educating the client about psychological constructs
- motivating the client
- helping the client to gain insight and to develop as a person
- improving the client's interpersonal relationships, coping ability, and building their resilience.

These worksheets can be used to enhance or guide treatment of a variety of problems, including:

- depression and mood disorders
- anxiety disorders, including generalised anxiety disorder, specific and social phobias, post-traumatic stress disorder, panic disorder, obsessive compulsive disorder, as well as worry and perfectionism
- anger and stress
- substance abuse
- interpersonal issues, including poor communication, bullying, lack of assertiveness, poor conflict resolution skills, inadequate social skills and low confidence
- low self-esteem, lack of direction and focus in life, lack of goal-achievement.

About the author

Dr Clare Rosoman (née Whiting) is a clinical psychologist currently managing a large not-for-profit psychology clinic in Queensland, Australia. Additionally, she is a consultant at Griffith University as a supervisor of postgraduate clinical psychology students in their work with clients. Clare received her Bachelor of Psychology with Honours from the University of New England and her Doctor of Psychology

(Clinical) from Griffith University in Brisbane, Australia. Since graduating she has worked in a variety of settings, including psychiatric hospitals, private practice, schools and universities. She is strongly interested in and has been active in the training of therapists such as psychologists, psychiatry registrars and general practitioners. She has had several papers published in the area of children's social functioning and antisocial behaviour.

She recognised a need for a resource for therapists that contained easy-to-use, simple worksheets from the fervour her students displayed in photocopying her folders of collected sheets. As a resource, this book represents years of accumulated therapy tools in one easy location. For training therapists, it provides security in the form of a tool-kit, and for more experienced therapists it avoids reinventing the wheel when a resource is needed for a session.

Acknowledgments

These activities and worksheets have been inspired by many theories and schools of thought in psychology, counselling and psychiatry. Many of the exercises draw from the principles of cognitive behavioural therapy (CBT), narrative therapy and solution-focused therapy, as well as the accumulated knowledge and wisdom of many practitioners. The author wishes to acknowledge the work of these amazing theorists and practitioners, and to emphasise that these worksheets represent a pooling of a vast wealth of shared knowledge and understanding in the practice of psychotherapy.

STARTERS

GETTING STARTED

1.1 Rapport building

The fundamental principle of a meaningful therapeutic relationship is rapport. If the client feels at ease with their therapist and can trust their therapist with their feelings, then therapy is given the utmost chance of being significant and productive.

This group of worksheets has been designed with this in mind. They range from simple 'getting to know you' sheets to more exploratory sheets for deeper disclosure. They all aim to put the client at ease, to build trust in the therapeutic relationship, and to allow the therapist to show an unconditional positive regard for the client.

Introducing ME!

This is a simple sheet designed to encourage non-threatening discussion about the client. This can be very useful in both group therapy, and individual therapy as it remains light and general while still allowing the therapist some insight into the client. It has a purely positive focus to create a feeling of safety and acceptance for the client and gives plenty of opportunities for the therapist to provide warmth and validation.

The Tree of Me

Ask the client to think about all the different parts of their life and to write these onto the branches of the tree. This could serve as a platform for deeper discussion about the roles they play in their life and how their difficulties change or affect these roles, and vice versa. The analogy of the tree lends itself to discussion about the association between 'branches' of the client's life, the relative weight of some of the branches, whether any of the branches are undernourished or have died, and what the client sees as their 'roots' in their life. This can lead to a deeper discussion about how well their 'tree' weathers storms and what nourishes and shelters it.

All about Me

This sheet encourages a deeper level of disclosure about the client. Therefore, it is more suitable for individual therapy and for clients who are comfortable with this level of discussion. It is valuable because it allows the therapist and the client to explore the deeper workings of the client, but always at the client's level of comfort.

Introducing ME!

My name is: _____

My star sign is: _____

Some of my favourite things are...

- favourite TV program: _____
- favourite food: _____
- favourite pastime: _____
- favourite holiday destination: _____

If I could be an animal I would be _____

because _____

_____

If I had a million dollars I would:

_____

Three things I am proud of:

_____

_____

_____

The Tree of Me

Write or draw some of the parts of you and your life onto the braches of the tree
e.g. family, hobbies, likes, dislikes, roles you play, sources of stress, etc.

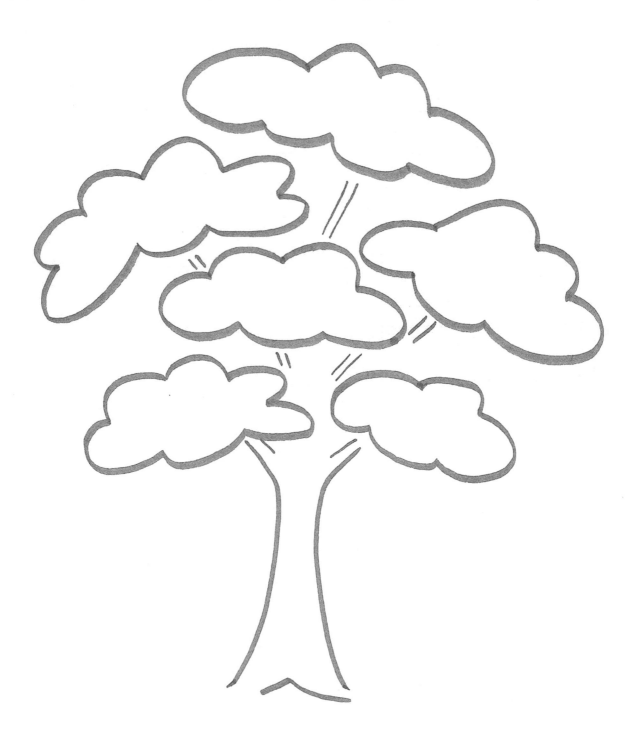

All about Me

When I think about who I really am _____

_____

_____

Growing up for me was _____

_____

_____

What I like about me is _____

_____

_____

Thinking into the future _____

_____

_____

Thinking about the past _____

_____

_____

All about Me *cont.*

People around me are _____

_____

_____

I wish _____

_____

_____

One day I would like to _____

_____

_____

Being me means _____

_____

_____

I wish people would _____

_____

_____

1.2 Boundaries

At the beginning of therapy it is important for the client to have a clear idea of the boundaries around the therapeutic relationship. For this to happen, they need to have a thorough understanding of confidentiality and its limits, of their personal safety and comfort in therapy, and of their own control over therapy and the treatment plan.

Confidentiality Form

This sheet has been compiled to clearly and simply explain confidentiality to the client. This is valuable to go through with your client in the early stages of the therapeutic relationship and could be used as an information sheet for clients at intake. Additionally, it might be useful to have this sheet presented in a visible location in your office.

Therapy...

This worksheet aims to extrapolate the client's feelings about coming to therapy and what it means for them to be there. It also allows the therapist to be apprised of any areas the client does not feel comfortable talking about so that the client is put at ease from the outset. This sheet empowers the client and allows them to feel in control of the therapeutic process. It allows for discussion should the client be reluctant to attend or if they have negative attributions relating to attending therapy. It also provides an opportunity for the therapist to explain about how they conduct therapy and to assure the client that all treatment goals will be collaborative.

Boundaries

This is an informative sheet used to describe the concept of boundaries. It uses a simple 'wall' analogy that can be extended to all relationships in the client's life, but particularly to explain that the therapeutic relationship is a special relationship, with the thickness of the wall being decided entirely by the client and their comfort level. It can also be used to set a clear boundary around the therapist by explaining that the wall for the client is thinner than the wall for the therapist, and that this is because it is a professional relationship for the client's benefit.

Confidentiality Form

Therapy is confidential

This means that information shared during therapy will be private and that all records are kept securely. I can only disclose information about our sessions *with your permission first*.

BUT...there are some exceptions

I am *obliged by law* to break confidentiality *without your permission* if:

- I am concerned that you may be a danger to yourself (deliberately harm yourself in any way)

- I am concerned that you may be a danger to others (deliberately harm another in any way)

- I am concerned that you may be going to do something illegal

- my records are subpoenaed by a court of law.

If I have to break confidentiality, *I will always try to tell you first*. Then, I am required to tell the appropriate authorities and to take the appropriate action.

Therapy...

How you feel about coming to therapy (*Mark the line where you fit*):

_____

Happy   positive   relieved   neutral   worried   angry   terrified

Words that come to mind about being here:

_____

Whose idea was it that you come to therapy?

_____

What would you like to work on in therapy?

_____

_____

Are there any things that you don't feel comfortable talking about in therapy?

_____

_____

What are your fears about therapy?

_____

_____

Boundaries

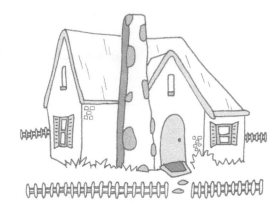

Boundaries are like an imaginary fence we all have around ourselves that define where our personal space begins and another's ends – like a fence around your house.

This sort of boundary is a **personal boundary** that determines how close you let others get to you (both physically and emotionally).

The boundary means that we **own ourselves** including our thoughts, feelings, beliefs, attitudes, choices, decisions, expectations, our body, dreams, goals, etc. If we had no boundaries, we would all get confused about what thoughts/beliefs/feelings belong to ourselves as opposed to others.

The closer you are to a person, the thinner, lower or more transparent your fence is with that person. This means that you let them closer to you **physically** (hugs/touching) and **emotionally** (share more of your feelings and innermost thoughts). For instance, you would have a thick boundary (brick wall) with someone you just met and would probably not share as much of yourself as you would with your mother (low wooden fence).

Who in your life do you have a very open boundary with? Who are you closest to of all the people in your life? Who knows the most about you?

_____

_____

_____

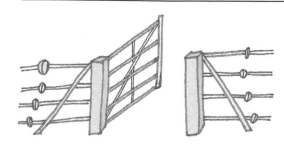

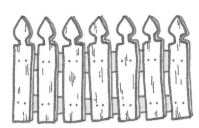

Who do you have a medium boundary with? Who knows some things about you but not everything?

_____

_____

_____

Who do you have a big, thick boundary with? Who do you never let in at all?

_____

_____

_____

1.3 Expectations for change

It is important to assess the client's expectations of therapy and their goals for change before proceeding into a treatment plan. Sometimes, the goals the therapist may have for a client do not match with the client's goals for themselves. Therefore, in the early stages of the therapeutic relationship, it is valuable to investigate this area. It is vital to hear the client's story and to show them that their needs and expectations are important to you as their therapist.

My Goals for Therapy

This worksheet asks the client to think of three things they would like to change in their lives through therapy and to rate their level of confidence in completing each goal. It gives the therapist an opportunity to assess the therapeutic goals from the perspective of the client and to also assess the client's expectations of themselves and of therapy. This means that from the outset of therapy, the therapist is completely aware of the client's expectations and can tailor the treatment plan to their needs. The client will also feel that they have been heard and included in the early stages of the relationship, and this will increase their investment in the therapy process.

Magic Wand

This is an unstructured approach to therapeutic goal-setting that can give startling insights into the client's life and expectations. It involves asking the client what they would change in their life if they had a magic wand. This can be used to any level of depth, thus it can warrant light, superficial information (non-threatening), particularly with the use of humour and the 'prop' of an actual wand, or can provide deeper discussion about the client's life situation.

My Life...

This sheet aims to investigate the client's current sources of stress and discomfort and to determine their attitude to those stressors. This allows the therapist to make a judgement about the client's level of self-efficacy and power in overcoming their obstacles. This gives valuable information about the client's readiness for therapy and their motivation for change.

My Goals for Therapy

Three things I would like to improve in myself or my life:

1. _____

_____

_____

Why? _____

_____

Rate your confidence in achieving this goal (circle):

1	2	3	4	5
Confident	Fairly confident	Unsure	Doubtful	Not confident

2. _____

_____

_____

Why? _____

_____

_____

My Goals for Therapy *cont.*

Rate your confidence in achieving this goal (circle):

1	2	3	4	5
Confident	Fairly confident	Unsure	Doubtful	Not confident

3. _____

_____

_____

Why? _____

_____

_____

Rate your confidence in achieving this goal (circle):

1	2	3	4	5
Confident	Fairly confident	Unsure	Doubtful	Not confident

Magic Wand

If you could wave a magic wand and change your life, what would you change? Write these things around the wand!

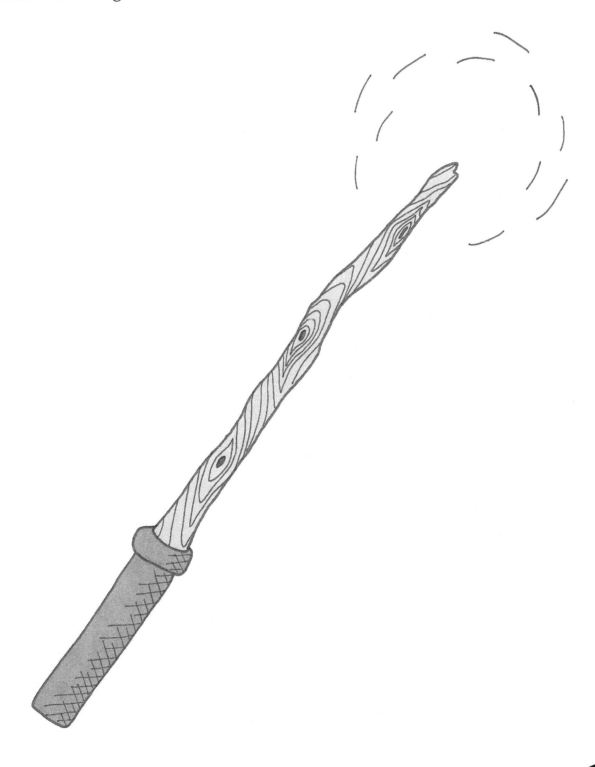

My Life...

My life is _____

I'm happiest when _____

I'm the most stressed when _____

I get frustrated by _____

No matter how hard I try I can't _____

When I think about me I feel _____

Ten years from now _____

The things that bother me the most are _____

I feel hopeless when _____

I feel positive about _____

1.4 Motivation for change

Launching into a treatment plan with a client who is not motivated to change is a disheartening experience for both the therapist and the client. More important, it can decrease the client's feeling of self-efficacy and control over their issues if they have a 'failure' to their credit. Many clients in this situation develop the belief that 'therapy doesn't work' and are reluctant to try in the future.

Therefore, it is important to assess the client's expectations of therapy and their motivation for change at an early stage, to make sure that the therapeutic goals are appropriate to their needs and are therefore likely to give them a feeling of success, no matter how small the goal. This will ensure that highly motivated clients are challenged and less motivated clients are given a positive experience of therapy and inspired to keep working on their bigger issues at a slower pace.

Putting the Boxing Gloves on

This sheet asks the client to list all the things that cause them distress in their life. It then asks them to rate out of ten the impact each issue has on their life, and their readiness to fight each issue. This allows the client to prioritise the stress in their life and to make an objective assessment of their readiness to tackle each issue. This makes it very clear for both parties which issues will be the easiest to target and which issues the client feels less confident about. This opens up discussion about motivation for change and personal power.

Things I have Control over and Things I don't...

Once the client has listed all of the things that cause them distress in their life (or spoken about those things with the therapist), it can be useful for them to reflect upon which stressors they feel they have control over and which things they feel they have no control over. This gives the therapist a useful insight into the client's issues and information about how best to empower the client to exercise more control over their life as a result of therapy. It also raises the important point that some things cannot be changed or controlled, and that therapy will need to focus on changing the client's reaction to those stressors rather than trying in vain to eradicate them.

Personal Power

In this exercise, the client is asked to think of two issues in their life and how powerful they feel in overcoming each issue. It also asks the client to reflect on prior situations when they may have beaten the issue, and what changes they are willing to make in order to tackle it. This leads to discussion about personal power, motivation and willingness to make changes in order to resolve an issue.

Narrative Therapy Questions

Narrative therapy takes a unique approach to therapy by externalising and naming the problem as an entity separate from the client. (For more information see M. White and D. Epston (1990), *Narrative Means to Therapeutic Ends*. New York, Norton.) This sheet is designed for use by the therapist in a dialogue with the client to explore a treatment-resistant presenting problem or to improve the client's motivation to confront an issue. The list of questions can be used in order or selected as appropriate.

Externalising the 'problem' and naming it (X) can sometimes allow a defensive or blocked client to align with the therapist against the problem, rather than seeing the problem as a fault within themselves. This approach can increase the client's awareness of warning signs, triggers, and the emotional and behavioural sequelae of the problem, all in a non-threatening manner. This can greatly improve motivation to manage and fight back against an issue.

Putting the Boxing Gloves on

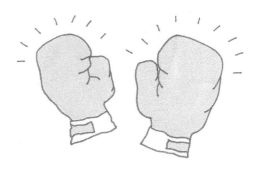

Things that cause me distress in my life	Level of impact
	Rate: 0–10
	  0 = *no impact*
	10 = *large impact*
		Readiness to fight
		Rate: 0–10
		  0 = *no impact*
		10 = *large impact*

Things I have Control over and Things I don't…

Divide the things that cause you distress in your life into two groups – those things you feel you have some control over and those things you feel you have no control over.

Things I feel I have some control over…

Things I don't feel I have control over…

Personal Power

Think of two issues in your life that you would like to change.

1. _____

a) Do you feel that you can overcome this issue if you put your mind to it? Why?

_____

_____

_____

b) Have you ever overcome this issue before? Why/how?

_____

_____

_____

c) What changes are you willing to make in order to tackle this issue?

_____

_____

_____

Personal Power *cont.*

2. _____

a) Do you feel that you can overcome this issue if you put your mind to it? Why?

_____

_____

_____

b) Have you ever overcome this issue before? Why/how?

_____

_____

_____

c) What changes are you willing to make in order to tackle this issue?

_____

_____

_____

Narrative Therapy Questions

What would you call the problem (X)?

How could you describe its characteristics?

How does it make you feel, think, behave?

How do you know when it is present in your life?

When do you see it sneaking up on you and how does it do that?

In what situations does it present itself?

What are the first signs within your body that tell you it is visiting?

How does it change how you act?

How does it affect your outlook on life?

Who are you with X?

Who are you without X?

Can you remember a time when X was not in your life? What was that like?

What does your future look like with X?

Do you like yourself better without X?

How has X changed your life? For the better or the worse?

How has X changed how you see the world?

How has X changed how you see yourself?

How has X changed who you are?

How has X changed how you treat others?

What parts of you have been unaffected by X? Why?

Do you feel that X has taken away or changed parts of you? Which parts and how?

Has there ever been a time when you have defeated X? What did you do? How did that feel?

What happens when X takes over?

Narrative Therapy Questions *cont.*

How can you fight X?

What tools do you have at your disposal to weaken X?

Do you want to fight X?

Do you feel strong enough to fight X?

What could you be free to do if X was not in your life?

What kind of person would you be without X?

What would your life be like without X?

What scares you about letting X go?

Are there any benefits to having X in your life?

How could you replace those benefits if you were to lose X?

1.5 Unfolding the story

Once the client understands the process and boundaries of therapy, the initial presenting problem has been discussed, and the client's expectations and motivation for change have been assessed, it is time to gather information about the client's history. This adds many layers to the presenting issue and helps in the development of rapport, the formulation or summary of the client's situation, and the subsequent treatment plan.

My Story

This sheet allows the client to tell their story in an unstructured manner, filling the page in any form they choose (e.g. writing, drawing, poetry, mind mapping, lifeline). Thus, this sheet allows for discriminating emphasis on the areas that they feel are most relevant. This gives the therapist information about the key areas of the client's life as nominated by them, therefore providing an opportunity for further discussion of areas included in the client's story and for obvious omissions to become apparent. It might help to photocopy and enlarge the page so that the client has plenty of room to record their story.

Personal History – Childhood Years

This is a more structured form that could be used as an intake form for the client to complete before their first session, or as a prompt for the therapist while conducting the intake interview with an adult client. There are three forms in this set that look at the client's history from three parts of their life. This form examines their childhood up until the age of 13.

Personal History – Adolescent Years

This is the second in the above set, and looks in detail at the client's adolescent period. It contains many questions to give the therapist a rounded view of the client's life during that time of their life. The questions may also serve as a prompt for the client to reflect upon their adolescent years.

Personal History – Adult Years

This is the third in the above set, and investigates the client's early adult years and onwards. For older clients, the therapist may have to improvise a little!

Making Sense of Things

This sheet allows the therapist to formulate the client's presenting problem by examining the factors that set the scene for the presenting problem (predisposing factors), the factors that brought it to a head currently or recently (precipitating factors) and the factors that are maintaining the presenting problem in the client's life (perpetuating factors). By presenting this to the client, this exercise is highly validating and helps to increase the client's insight into their issues. This then prepares the client for treatment and allows the therapist to present their rationale for treatment (how it will address the maintaining factors and work through predisposing and precipitating factors). This is best completed by the therapist and fed back to the client or done collaboratively in session.

Reflecting on the Past

This is a structured worksheet that could be a reflective task for a homework activity or for a directed discussion in session to help the client to reflect on their past and to gain insight into their issues. This helps the therapist to understand the client and their history and to detect any patterns that may be contributing to the presenting complaint.

My Story

Personal History – Childhood Years

Describe your family life when you were aged 0–13:

_____

_____

What is your earliest childhood memory?

_____

_____

How many siblings do/did you have? What are their names and order of birth?

_____

_____

Describe your relationship with your siblings:

_____

_____

What was your relationship like with your mother?

_____

_____

What was your relationship like with your father?

_____

_____

Describe your experiences at primary school (including academic and social aspects):

_____

_____

What are your best and worst memories from primary school?

_____

_____

Did the presenting problem begin in childhood? If so, how?

_____

_____

Personal History – Adolescent Years

What was your family life like during your adolescent years (13–18)?

_____

_____

Did your relationship change with your parents during this time of your life? How?

_____

_____

What was your relationship like with your siblings?

_____

_____

Who were your best friends? Describe them?

_____

_____

What were your favourite pastimes?

_____

_____

What did you get in trouble for?

_____

_____

Describe your experiences at high school (including academic and social aspects):

_____

_____

What worried or upset you as a teenager? Why?

_____

_____

What are your best and worst memories from adolescence?

_____

_____

Did your presenting problem begin in adolescence or change during this time? How?

_____

_____

Personal History – Adult Years

What has happened in your life since the age of 18 to the present?

_____

_____

_____

What types of study and/or employment have you undertaken?

_____

_____

_____

Describe any significant long-term relationships you have had (including children):

_____

_____

_____

What difficulties would you like help with by coming here?

_____

_____

_____

How have these problems developed or changed in your adult years?

_____

_____

_____

What have been your saddest and proudest moments in your adulthood?

_____

_____

_____

Are you currently taking any medications? (list names and dosages)

_____

_____

_____

Has anyone in your family suffered from mental health issues?

_____

_____

_____

Making Sense of Things

The main issues that are disrupting your life are:

⇩

The factors that set the scene for the development of these issues are:

⇩

The factors that set it off or brought it to a head are:

⇩

The factors that are maintaining these difficulties are:

Reflecting on the Past

When I think about the past I feel...

The things I am most proud of...

The things that have had the most impact on me are...

The people I have learned from are...

Three things I would change...

Where I see my journey going in the future...

2 THERAPY BASICS

2.1 Exploring and expressing emotions

Talking about feelings forms a major part of the therapeutic process. Consequently, this section contains a variety of worksheets to assist clients in their interpretation and naming of emotions and in their deeper understanding of their feelings and reactions to the world.

Emotions List

This sheet lists many of the emotions experienced by all people. Such an exhaustive list can aid in the identification of feelings by providing a wide range of examples.

Emotions

This sheet asks some broad questions about emotions to elicit some thought about their advantages and disadvantages. The aim is for the client to understand that emotions are important because without them we would have no measure of our lives: what is normal, what is great, what is bad, what is dangerous. The therapist may need to guide the client to understand that emotions are negative when they are *inappropriate to a situation* (e.g. laughing at a funeral), when they are *too intense* (eg. extreme anger, sadness or anxiety), when they are *uncomfortable* (eg. cause negative symptoms – heart palpitations, headaches, nausea, sleep loss), and when they *stop you from feeling good about yourself or from achieving your goals.*

Understanding Emotions

This sheet allows the client to analyse one emotion that causes them difficulty in their life and to increase their awareness of their body's reaction to it, when it is helpful and unhelpful, and the things that trigger it. This is intended to increase the client's awareness and motivation to challenge the emotion.

My Feelings

This worksheet can be worked through in session or for homework and encourages the client to think about their feelings and their impact on their life. It can provide the therapist with valuable information regarding the most prominent emotions causing problems for the client. This also helps the client to objectively review the emotions that cause them the most difficulty.

What are Emotions?

This is a psycho-educational worksheet that aims to explain the many facets of emotions. It begins by explaining why we have emotions and then explains that all emotions contain cognitive (thoughts), behavioural and physiological (body's reaction) elements. Two examples are provided and then the client is encouraged to look at a third emotion and to break it down into its components. This sheet paves the way for the introduction of the cognitive model by introducing the client to the cognitive and behavioural components of emotion.

Expressing Feelings

This activity aims to increase clients' awareness of the verbal and nonverbal components of four emotions. It is especially useful for adults with limited emotional understanding, particularly regarding the nonverbal elements of emotions. It is often very validating for the client to understand the complexity of emotions because it helps them to understand why emotions can cause such havoc in peoples' lives. This exercise can increase emotional awareness with a view to moving on to emotional regulation training. It can also provide a foundation for communication skills training by helping clients to be aware of the nonverbal make-up of emotion and the way they express these emotions to others.

Emotions List

 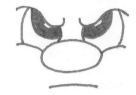 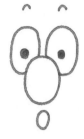 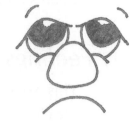

aggressive	angry	alienated	alone	annoyed
bored	cautious	confident	confused	curious
discouraged	disgusted	embarrassed	disappointed	enthusiastic
excited	exhausted	fearful	frightened	frustrated
happy	helpless	hopeful	hostile	humiliated
innocent	interested	jealous	joyful	jumpy
loved	loving	mischievous	miserable	negative
paranoid	peaceful	proud	puzzled	regretful
sorry	shocked	shy	satisfied	stubborn
surprised	suspicious	thoughtful	undecided	withdrawn
unmotivated	pessimistic	black	flat	numb
turbulent	energetic	terrified	independent	needy
wary	cooperative	relaxed	scared	brave
affectionate	steady	inhibited	isolated	repelled
agitated	evasive	turmoil	secure	pained
avoidant	insecure	lethargic	sad	lonely
ecstatic	determined	apathetic	grief	hysterical
impulsive	vindictive	lacklustre	anguished	jittery
indignant	safe	relieved	optimistic	hurt
guilty	envious	depressed	anxious	placid

Emotions

Why do we have them?

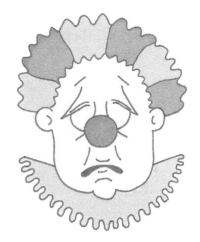

When are they positive?

When are they negative?

Understanding Emotions

One emotion that causes me difficulty is: _____
Draw onto the person all the physical feelings related to your emotion, e.g. tight chest, tense muscles, or low energy, etc.

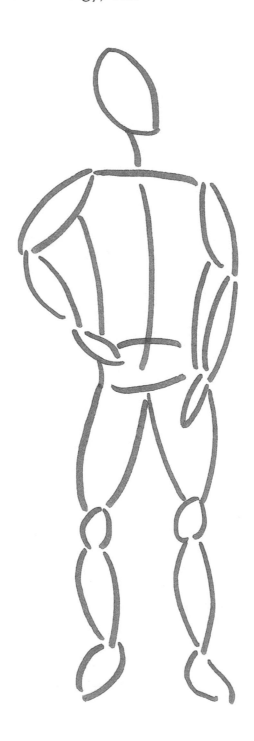

When is this emotion helpful and why?

When is it unhelpful and why?

What things usually happen that cause this emotion?

My Feelings

I am happiest when _____

I get scared when _____

I am confused by _____

I feel guilty when _____

I am hurt by _____

I am embarrassed by _____

I am envious of _____

I feel sad when _____

I am frustrated by _____

What are Emotions?

Emotions are complex reactions to our world that act as a 'warning system' allowing us to interpret our surroundings, communicate with others, and keep ourselves safe.

Emotional reactions are made up of three parts:

1. **Thoughts:** what you say to yourself.

2. **Behaviours:** what you do when experiencing that emotion.

3. **Our body's physiological reaction:** the changes that happen in your body as a result of that emotion.

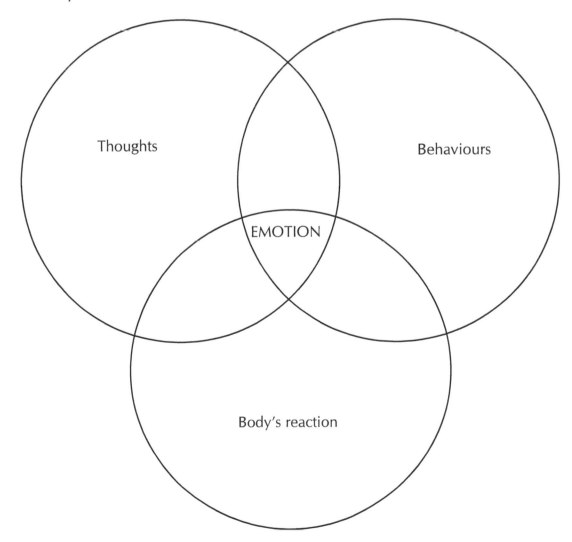

What are Emotions? *cont.*

As an example, let's look at the emotion of ANXIETY:

1. **Thoughts:** 'Oh no, I'm really scared, I can't cope!'

2. **Behaviours:** running away, avoiding, putting things off.

3. **Body's reaction:** sweating, shaking, nausea, rapid heart rate.

Another example: the emotion of SADNESS:

1. **Thoughts:** 'Nothing ever will work out for me.'

2. **Behaviours:** crying, isolation, stop trying.

3. **Body's reaction:** lethargy, appetite changes, sleep disturbance.

Now you try one! Pick an emotion _____

1. **Thoughts:** _____

2. **Behaviours:** _____

3. **Body's reaction:** _____

Expressing Feelings

We use a variety of words, phrases and actions to express feelings. This exercise aims to help you explore the ways we show emotion.

For each of the following feelings, write down the words, phrases, tone of voice and actions that you could use to express them.

HAPPINESS
Words
Phrases
Tone of voice
Actions

ANXIETY/FEAR
Words
Phrases
Tone of voice
Actions

ANGER
Words
Phrases
Tone of voice
Actions

SADNESS
Words
Phrases
Tone of voice
Actions

2.2 Monitoring

It is important for the therapist to gain reliable data about the client's life in order to set appropriate treatment goals and to assess the progress of therapy. Additionally, it is essential that the client learns to collect evidence about their difficulty in order for them to see changes, to challenge their beliefs, and to maintain a realistic and scientific approach to their issue. To aid in this process, this group of monitoring sheets has been collected.

Feelings Thermometer

This chart illustrates for the client a ten-point scale for monitoring emotion. It is a useful tool because it creates a common language between the therapist and the client about the intensity of emotions, as well as providing an objective scale for the client to learn to rate their emotions on.

Daily Mood Log

This monitoring sheet asks the client to record their mood on three different occasions throughout the day. The aim of this form is to increase the client's understanding of their feelings and the triggers (antecedents) for them. This prepares the client for therapy by increasing their awareness of their 'activating events'.

Monitoring Mood

This is a very simple mood monitoring sheet that increases clients' awareness of their moods throughout a day by asking them to name and rate their mood/feeling out of ten and to reflect upon what may have contributed to that emotional state, as well as what they did in response. It aims to collect valuable information for the therapist regarding the client's emotional state, as well as increasing the client's awareness of their feelings and their triggers.

Monitoring a Target Behaviour

This monitoring form focuses on a target behaviour that the client is hoping to reduce during therapy. It involves the client recording on the table each time they engage in the target behaviour. It also requires the client to think about the triggers for their behaviour and to record anything they may have done to try to prevent the target behaviour or to reduce its impact. This provides the therapist and the client with a baseline in order to commence treatment.

Linking Feelings, Behaviour and Thoughts

This monitoring sheet is slightly more advanced as it asks the client to record their behaviours and thoughts at the time that they experienced a negative emotion. This sheet is best used when a target emotion has been identified and the therapist aims to increase the client's insight into the behaviours and thoughts associated with that emotion. It particularly encourages the client to identify the effect of emotions on behaviours and vice versa.

Feelings Thermometer

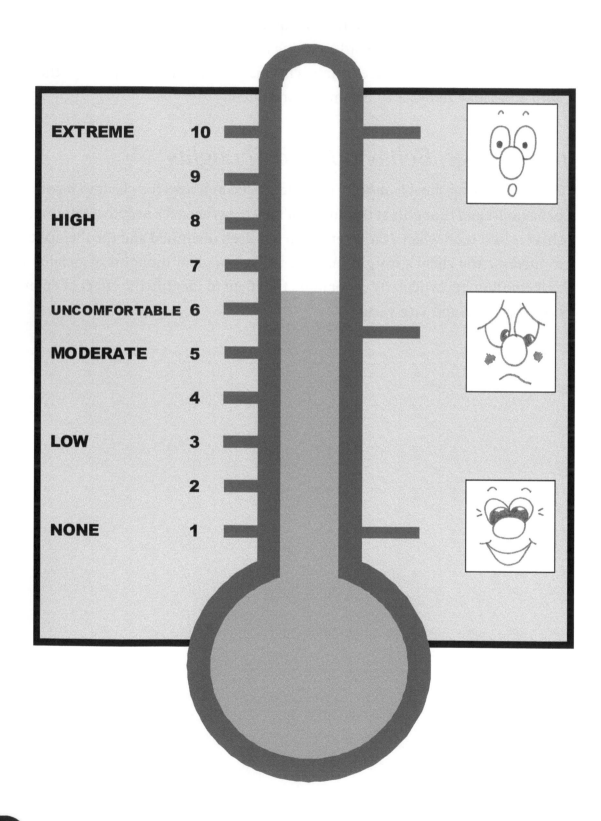

EXTREME 10

9

HIGH 8

7

UNCOMFORTABLE 6

MODERATE 5

4

LOW 3

2

NONE 1

Daily Mood Log

Day: _____   **Date:** _____

Morning
My emotion: _____   **Rating (0–10):** _____

What happened before I felt like this? _____

_____

_____

Did this cause my emotion? If not, what did? _____

_____

_____

Midday
My emotion: _____   **Rating (0–10):** _____

What happened before I felt like this? _____

_____

_____

Daily Mood Log *cont.*

Did this cause my emotion? If not, what did? _____

_____

_____

Evening

My emotion: _____   **Rating (0–10):** _____

What happened before I felt like this? _____

_____

_____

Did this cause my emotion? If not, what did? _____

_____

_____

Monitoring Mood

Record on the table each time you notice a change in your mood or feelings throughout the day.

Day: _____   **Date:** _____

Mood	Rate out of 10	What happened? What caused this feeling? What did you do in response?

Monitoring a Target Behaviour

Record on the table each time you engage in your target behaviour throughout the day.

Target behaviour that you want to reduce: _____

Day: _____   **Date:** _____

Behaviour (what you did)	What happened? What triggered this behaviour? What did you do to try to prevent it?

Linking Feelings, Behaviour and Thoughts

What are you feeling (0–10)? _____

What is your behaviour? _____

Thoughts (What are you telling yourself?)	What happened first? (What set it off?)	What was the result of your behaviour?

What are you feeling (0–10)? _____

What is your behaviour? _____

Thoughts (What are you telling yourself?)	What happened first? (What set it off?)	What was the result of your behaviour?

Linking Feelings, Behaviour and Thoughts *cont.*

What are you feeling (0–10)? _____

What is your behaviour? _____

Thoughts (What are you telling yourself?)	What happened first? (What set it off?)	What was the result of your behaviour?

What are you feeling (0–10)? _____

What is your behaviour? _____

Thoughts (What are you telling yourself?)	What happened first? (What set it off?)	What was the result of your behaviour?

2.3 Cognitive behavioural therapy (CBT)

This section aims to present some of the main ideas and techniques of cognitive behavioural therapy in worksheet format for the client. (For more information see Judith Beck (1995) *Cognitive Therapy: Basics and Beyond*. New York: Guilford Press.) Although the concepts of CBT are readily digestible and clear to the therapist, sometimes it can take the client some time to assimilate all the information. As a result, psycho-educational information sheets and homework sheets can be extremely useful.

What is CBT?

This worksheet aims to demystify CBT for the client by explaining it clearly and simply. Having a good understanding of the therapeutic rationale can greatly increase a client's motivation to commit to therapy. When the client understands why the therapist is asking them to complete an activity (particularly if it is uncomfortable), they are far more likely to attempt it and to give it their best effort. Therefore, this sheet forms an introduction to the techniques of CBT and the concepts behind them.

The Workings of Emotions

This sheet builds on the 'What are Emotions?' sheet on page 55 in Section 2.1. It explains the role of thinking and perception in emotional and behavioural reactions. This lays a foundation for the challenging of unhelpful thoughts later in this section and clearly conveys the message that it is not our world that determines our emotions but rather, our perception of that world.

Recording your Thoughts

This sheet provides space for the client to practice identifying the events that lead to a negative emotion and/or behaviour. This helps them to clearly differentiate between thoughts, emotions and behaviours and to see the powerful effect of thinking on emotions and behaviours.

Challenging your Thoughts

This is a list of questions the client can ask themselves to help them to challenge their unhelpful thoughts. This prepares the client to construct more realistic and helpful thoughts to replace the unhelpful ones. These could then be made into a poster or put on to coping cards for the client to carry with them.

Changing your Thinking

This sheet gives the client space to write in their unhelpful thoughts and to challenge them with the questions in the previous worksheet before coming up with a more helpful alternative thought. This sheet can be used as the basis for deeper cognitive therapy and is a very useful homework sheet. The more clients practice this technique by completing this sheet, the more the process of cognitive restructuring becomes habit. This exercise is invaluable in teaching clients to 'catch' their unhelpful thoughts and to challenge and change them into more helpful and adaptive thoughts.

Digging Deep

This sheet aims to uncover the deeper or 'core' beliefs behind a client's surface-level, automatic thoughts. This is a meaningful exercise that provides deep insights into the development and maintenance of maladaptive patterns of unhelpful thinking. This can be completed with the therapist or individually to increase insight. Often, cognitive restructuring is ineffective when the deeper, core beliefs go unchallenged. Therefore, this exercise can be instrumental in uncovering blocks, vulnerabilities and innermost fears. Being able to challenge and dispute these deeper beliefs can begin the process of weakening them and so reducing their impact upon the automatic or surface-level thoughts that affect a client's everyday functioning.

What is CBT?

- Cognitive behavioural therapy (CBT) is a type of therapy that focuses on the role of thinking and behaviour in emotion.

- It was originally developed by American psychiatrist Aaron T. Beck who maintained that the way you think and behave greatly affects your emotions. He introduced the approach in *Depression: Causes and Treatment* (1967). His ideas have been developed and expanded by many others and the effectiveness of CBT has been proven repeatedly in research.

- Therefore, the basis of CBT is that **you can change the way you think and behave to change the way you feel**.

How do you do that?

- **First**, you need to become aware of your thoughts, feelings and behaviours and the *difference* between them:

  - **thoughts:** what you tell yourself (in words) in your mind.

  - **feelings:** emotions you experience (angry, sad, fearful, happy etc.)

  - **behaviours:** things you do or your body does (eg. sweating, avoiding, hiding, yelling, running away, crying, tensing up, smiling).

- **Second**, you need to be clear about *which* feelings and behaviours create problems for you that you want to change.

- **Third**, you need to pay close attention to the *thoughts* you tell yourself when you experience those negative emotions or behaviours.

- **Finally**, CBT teaches you to challenge your thoughts and to replace the unhelpful ones with more helpful, realistic thoughts. These realistic thoughts will help you to reduce the levels of negative or inappropriate emotions you experience.

- **Additionally**, you will learn different behaviours to help change the way you feel and to help you feel more positive in general.

An example:

John was a postman who often delivered letters to houses with barking dogs. He had been bitten by a dog as a child and had developed a fear of all dogs ever since. John decided he needed to overcome his fear of dogs when he realised that his level of fear was stopping him from working productively.

In his CBT, he learned first to differentiate between his thoughts, feelings and behaviours and to look at his beliefs about dogs. He realised that his thoughts were very extreme and that they were creating his high level of fear. He had convinced himself that *every* barking dog was a threat to his safety.

CBT taught him to think in a more realistic way about the threat of being bitten and to challenge himself to face his fear by going to all the houses with barking dogs to deliver mail. He learned to relax his body and to calm his mind in order to think more clearly and rationally. By doing this, he proved his fears wrong and decreased his level of anxiety. This caused him to feel more confident and to perform better in his job.

The Workings of Emotions

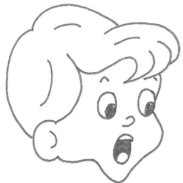

Emotions are complex reactions to our world that are made up of thoughts, physical responses and behaviours.

For example, the emotion of anxiety is felt through our **body's reaction** (i.e. tension, heart racing, sweating, shaking), our **behaviours** (talking fast, hiding, running away, agitation), and our **thoughts** (fearful, negative and catastrophic: *Oh no, I can't cope!*).

What affects our emotions?

Most people think that events in their world directly cause their emotional reactions. However, this is not true. It is how we **perceive** events in our world through our thoughts that really determines our reactions to those events.

Our thoughts act as a filter to our world and as a gatekeeper between our world and our reactions. If we did not all perceive our worlds differently, we would all have identical reactions.

It is our life experiences that shape our thoughts and perceptions of our world – which, in turn, shape our emotional and behavioural reactions to our world.

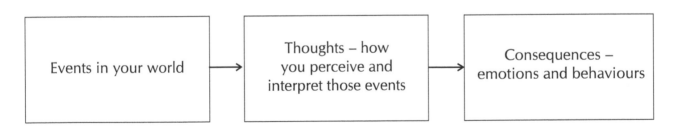

This means that if a person experiences a very negative emotional and behavioural reaction to something in their life (to which others don't react so negatively), then they need to examine their thoughts and beliefs about that part of their life in order to understand their negative reaction.

Cognitive behavioural therapy is the process of **changing unhelpful thoughts and behaviours** so that the negative emotion reduces in intensity.

Recording your Thoughts

Event What happened? e.g. friend broke her promise.	Thoughts What you actually told yourself. e.g. 'I can't believe she did that!'	Emotions Name and rate (0–10). e.g. angry (8) and anxious (6)	Behaviour Describe what you did or your body did. e.g. I yelled and my heart rate increased.

Challenging your Thoughts

Once you have identified the thoughts behind a negative or inappropriate emotion you are experiencing, it is time to examine how realistic and helpful those thoughts are. Use the list below to challenge your unhelpful thoughts:

- **Am I exaggerating?**

- **Am I making things out to be worse than they really are?**

- **Am I sure this is really going to happen?**

- **Does it really matter what other people think?**

- **Is this really true?**

- **Am I forgetting the positives?**

- **Can I expect to be perfect in everything I do?**

- **Am I being fair to myself?**

- **Can I be expected to be right every time?**

- **Is it the end of the world?**

- **Have I survived this before?**

- **Do I have any experiences that prove that this thought is not true?**

- **If someone else thought this way, what would you say to them?**

- **Am I blaming myself for something that is not in my control?**

- **What is the worst that could happen and how likely is it?**

Changing your Thinking

Event: _____

Behaviour: _____

Emotions (0–10): _____

Thoughts	Challenge	Alternative thought
What you actually told yourself	Pick a challenge question from the 'Challenging your Thoughts' list for each thought – answer back to your thought!	A more helpful and realistic thought

How do you feel now?
Emotions (0–10):

Digging Deep

Use this table to uncover the deeper beliefs behind your surface-level 'automatic' thoughts. See if you can get to the bottom of the left column, then go back and challenge each level of your thoughts.

Unhelpful, automatic thought	Emotion	Helpful, realistic thought	Emotion
If that were true, what would that mean for you?			
If that were true, what would that mean for you?			
If that were true, what would that mean for you?			
If that were true, what would that mean for you?			
If that were true, what would that mean for you?			

2.4 Emotional regulation

This section contains activities that help the client to understand their emotions and to feel more in control of any negative or self-destructive emotional states that they may experience. This is especially important for clients who feel overwhelmed by their negative emotions and who sometimes engage in maladaptive behaviours when acutely emotional (e.g. self-harm, substance abuse, eating issues). It is important that these clients learn skills to manage their negative emotions before the therapist encourages them to expose their deeper feelings.

Triggers and Warning Signs

This exercise takes the client through one particular problematic emotion and explores its early warning signs and triggers. This increases the client's insight into their negative emotion and makes it seem more manageable and less threatening. This then provides a clear direction for the treatment plan and will hopefully motivate the client to challenge themselves. The earlier the client intervenes to prevent the escalation of an unhelpful emotion, the better.

Links in the Chain

This worksheet guides the client through the process of breaking down a problem behaviour into its many parts. It looks at the specific triggers for the problem behaviour and the consequences of that behaviour (both positive and negative). The aim of this sheet is to help the client to intercept with a more adaptive coping response anywhere along this chain to prevent the problem behaviour from occurring or the negative consequences from occurring. This forms a sound framework for the treatment goals and helps the client to see the importance of early intervention.

Staying in Control

This sheet lists some different ways for clients to stay in control of their emotions, particularly if they know that they can become destructive when their emotions escalate. The aim is for their awareness to increase (using the previous two worksheets) and for them to replace maladaptive behaviours with more helpful and constructive behaviours from the list. There is space for the client and therapist to add other helpful behaviours to this list. This sheet greatly increases the client's motivation to stay in control of their negative emotions by providing practical strategies for coping.

Crisis Plan

This crisis plan provides an opportunity for the client and the therapist to discuss safety, suicidal ideation and self-harm in a solution-focused manner. It prepares the vulnerable client with a list of contact numbers that they can use should they need to. The numbers that the therapist puts in the 'professional' categories will depend upon the therapist's model of therapy, the workplace and the expectations of that therapist. For example, some therapists provide the numbers of crisis agencies for 24-hour phone counselling, and others give the client a phone number to contact them in an emergency.

Triggers and Warning Signs

Which emotion causes the most problems for you?

How and why does this emotion cause you problems?

What physical feelings do you first notice when this emotion is starting to appear (e.g. tense muscles, tight chest, heart pounding, sweating, sick in the stomach, want to cry, etc.)

THIS IS YOUR EARLY WARNING SIGN!!

What things usually set this emotion off in your life (e.g. fighting with a friend, sitting an exam, going to a party, public speaking, job interviews)

THESE ARE YOUR TRIGGERS!!

Now that you have identified the things that **trigger** this unhelpful emotion and your **early warning signs**, you have taken a huge step in beating it! **Catch it early** and do something to **reduce it** before it grows!

Links in the Chain

What is the **PROBLEM BEHAVIOUR** I want to *reduce*?

What are the things in *my environment* that **TRIGGER** this behaviour?

What are the things *within me* that **TRIGGER** this behaviour?

What are my **EARLY WARNING SIGNS** that I am about to engage in this behaviour?

What are the **CONSEQUENCES** for *me* if I engage in this behaviour?

What are the **CONSEQUENCES** for *others* if I engage in this behaviour?

What are some ways I can reduce the **TRIGGERS** in my *environment*?

What are some ways I can reduce the **TRIGGERS** within *myself*?

What are some of the **POSITIVE CONSEQUENCES** of reducing this behaviour?

Staying in Control

Below are some suggestions to help you stay in control when you feel unsafe, upset or just a bit vulnerable.

- Talk to someone.

- Take some time out in a calm, quiet place.

- Write your thoughts down on paper.

- Exercise to burn off energy.

- Listen to restful or positive music.

- Be around people who make you feel more positive and safe.

- Immerse yourself in nature, concentrate on the smells, sounds and textures – lie on the grass, sit on the beach, go bushwalking.

- Breathe slowly, smoothly and calmly – say to yourself 'in-two-three-pause-out-two-three' as you breathe. Slow each breath down.

- Distract yourself in the short term with a movie, TV, talking to others or by being busy, then come back to the problem when you are calmer.

- Remind yourself that this feeling will pass and that you can cope.

- Delay any action that you want to do but know is not good for you by 10 minutes, then another 10 minutes, until the urge passes.

- Make a list of 'feel-good strategies' that help you to feel better, and stick it up on your wall. Pick one and do it immediately.

Can you think of any others?
•
•
•

Crisis Plan

This plan is to be used whenever you feel acutely unsafe or at risk of doing something destructive towards yourself or someone else.

Who I can call

FAMILY MEMBER: Phone:

FAMILY MEMBER: Phone:

PROFESSIONAL: Phone:

PROFESSIONAL: Phone:

FRIEND: Phone:

FRIEND: Phone:

What I can do

-
-
-

Other important numbers

- Emergency services (police, ambulance, fire):

-

-

2.5 Goal-setting

This section concentrates on goal-setting by looking at what goals are and why we have them, how to set a goal, and ways to motivate your client to achieve their goals. The sheets are practical and self-explanatory but can greatly help the client to be motivated and focused throughout the therapy process.

What's in a Goal?

This is an information sheet about the importance of goals and how to set goals. It could be used as a basis for discussion or given as a homework exercise along with a 'My Goal' sheet (see below). It provides a structured, step-by-step guide to goal-setting.

How to Achieve your Goals

This is another information sheet about goal-setting but this sheet focuses on how to motivate oneself to achieve goals once they have been set. This is particularly valuable if clients report that they procrastinate in getting started on their goals or if they feel discouraged and give up before they achieve their goals. This sheet provides useful tips and strategies to deal with both of these difficulties.

Unrealistic Goals

This is an educational sheet about unrealistic goal-setting and the motivations behind it. It explores three types of unrealistic goal-setting including, vague, perfectionistic and artificial goals. This sheet might help the therapist raise these issues with a client who seems to be falling into these traps.

My Goal

This sheet guides the client through the process of goal-setting. It is a fairly detailed format for more complex goals that require more in-depth planning. This gives the therapist a chance to coach the client in good goal-setting habits. Once the client understands this process, this can be a useful homework sheet to encourage the client to set, plan and monitor their own goals.

Personal Goals

In this exercise, the client has room to plan four goals in less detail than the last sheet. This is likely to suit clients with less complex goals. It is a less threatening sheet that is quick and easy to use.

Goal for the Day, Week, Month

This sheet asks clients to think of short-term and longer-term goals. Its simple format makes it non-threatening and ideal for sticking up on the wall to prompt continued work on the goals. It also demonstrates to the client that in order to achieve their longer-term goals, they need to begin working on them each day.

My Five-year Plan

This plan questions the client about various aspects of their life that they might want to change within the next five years. This sheet can be used to help clients to find direction and focus in their life and to think about where they are heading. It forces them to reflect upon the things that really matter to them and to look at the small steps they could start taking now to work towards their larger goals.

Determining my Life Goals

This sheet provides an opportunity for a detailed examination of the client's life and their dreams and goals. It includes eight aspects of a person's life and encourages the client to turn dreams into goals that can be tackled one by one. This gives the therapist insight into the deeper dreams and desires of the client.

What's in a Goal?

A goal is something that gives you direction and focus for the future. It gives you something to aim for and helps you to get what you want from your life.

Goals can have lots of positive benefits

- Goals motivate you.
- They help you to feel satisfied with your life and yourself.
- They give you purpose and direction.
- Goals help you to get what you want.
- Having a goal makes your life interesting.
- Goals provide you with a challenge.
- Goals can help to push you out of your comfort zone.
- By achieving a goal, you can surprise yourself at your capabilities.
- Completing a goal gives you a sense of pride and satisfaction.
- Having goals helps you to feel in control of your life.

How do you set goals?

1. **THINK** carefully about *what* you want to achieve (not what others want you to achieve!) and *why* – what's in it for you?

2. **DEFINE** your goal in words. State what it is that you *will* do, not what you *won't* do. Be positive about your goal.

3. Be **PRECISE** about your goal. Define exactly what it is that you plan to do. Clear goals are easier to achieve.

4. Be **REALISTIC** when setting your goal. A small manageable goal is more likely to be successful. Success increases self-esteem.

5. Break your goal down into **SMALL STEPS** so that each step is a reasonable size.

6. **PRIORITISE** your goals. Work on the most important ones first.

7. Remember to be **FLEXIBLE** with your goal; be prepared to modify it if you need to.

How to Achieve your Goals

Once you have set a goal for yourself, it can be hard to find the motivation to get started and to keep working at it until you complete it. Here are some suggestions to help you stay motivated in your goal achievement.

If you can't get started:

- break it down into smaller steps
- prioritise your goals and start the most important one first
- begin with the first step and do it straight away!
- use problem-solving to find out why you can't get started
- is the goal really something you want?
- look at what is stopping you and try to remove those obstacles
- remember why you wanted to achieve the goal in the first place
- write the goal down and stick it up where you will see it every day!
- do something every day towards your goal.

If you can't finish it:

- break the remainder of the goal down into smaller, more manageable steps
- be prepared to alter the goal or the deadline – give yourself more time to achieve it if you need to
- use problem-solving to look at why you are finding it hard to achieve the goal
- is the goal still important to you? Have your needs or priorities changed?
- are there other pressures on you that need addressing first?
- look at what is stopping you and try to remove those obstacles
- remember why you wanted to achieve the goal in the first place
- if you need to, set yourself a deadline – sometimes a bit of pressure helps us all!

Unrealistic Goals

Unrealistic goals are:

Vague	Perfectionistic	Artificial
No clear steps or deadline. No direction or purpose.	Unattainable, unrealistic and disappointing.	Not your own goals, things you think you *should* do.

What is behind unrealistic goal-setting?

Negative thinking!

Believing:	Believing:	Believing:
'I won't achieve it anyway.' 'Nothing ever works out for me.' 'Why bother?' 'It's not worth it.' 'It's too hard.' 'I don't know where to start.' 'I don't know what I want.' 'I need to worry about everyone else.'	'If I set a goal, I have to do it perfectly or not at all.' 'I will fail if I can't do it perfectly.' 'If it's not done perfectly, it's not worth doing.' 'I must be perfect in everything I do.' 'I don't do things in half measures.' 'I can't make a mistake.' 'I'll just wait until I can do it perfectly before I start.'	'I should do this because it will make my family proud of me.' 'All people should do...' 'To be a mature person I should be doing...' 'I don't know what I want.' 'I want to make others proud of me.' 'I don't want to be a disappointment.' 'If I just do this, I will feel better about myself.'

My Goal

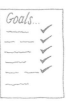

My goal: _____

_____

Why I want to achieve this goal: _____

_____

Step 1: _____

Step 2: _____

Step 3: _____

Step 4: _____

What do I need to achieve this goal (help, time, materials etc.)? _____

_____

What may interfere with my achievement of this goal? _____

_____

Solutions to these problems: _____

_____

When would I like to have this goal achieved? _____

Personal Goals

GOAL 1 _____

_____

Step 1: _____

_____

Step 2: _____

_____

Step 3: _____

_____

Step 4: _____

_____

GOAL 2 _____

_____

Step 1: _____

_____

Step 2: _____

_____

Step 3: _____

_____

Step 4: _____

_____

GOAL 3 _____

_____

Step 1: _____

_____

Step 2: _____

_____

Step 3: _____

_____

Step 4: _____

_____

GOAL 4 _____

_____

Step 1: _____

_____

Step 2: _____

_____

Step 3: _____

_____

Step 4: _____

_____

Goal for the Day

My goal for the **day** is: _____

_____

_____

_____

Goal for the Week

My goal for the **week** is: _____

_____

_____

_____

Goal for the Month

My goal for the **month** is: _____

_____

_____

My Five-year Plan

Imagine your life in five years' time...

What would you like to be achieving in your family life? _____

_____

_____

_____

What would you like to be achieving in your work life? _____

_____

_____

_____

What would you like to be achieving in your social life? _____

_____

_____

_____

What would you like to be achieving in your lifestyle (health, hobbies, etc.)?

_____

_____

_____

What would you like to achieve in terms of your self-development? _____

_____

_____

_____

Do you have any other goals that you would like to have achieved in five years' time?

_____

_____

_____

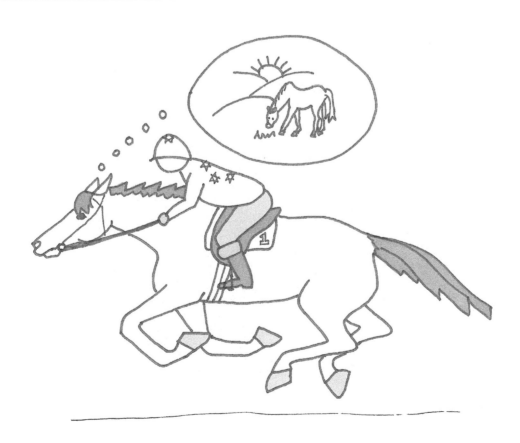

Determining my Life Goals

Life areas Areas of your life in which you might want to develop, change or improve.	Dreams and wants What you would like to change, improve or develop about these areas of your life.	Goals Turning these dreams and wants into realistic, specific, attainable goals. They can then be broken down into steps.
Family life		
Social life		
Career		
Hobbies and recreation		
Learning		
Health		
Personal development		
Other		
Other		

2.6 Problem-solving

This section provides some different exercises to help guide the client through the process of problem-solving and decision-making. These worksheets make excellent homework tasks, supply stimulus for discussion, and shape the client's coping skills.

Steps to Problem-solving

This is an information sheet that outlines the theory behind problem-solving. It can be used with the following problem-solving sheet or as an educational sheet to be used as a rough guide for the client in solving a problem. It provides clear steps that guide the client to define the problem, weigh up all their options and select and plan the best solution for them.

Problem-solving

This is a blank sheet that guides the client through the steps of problem-solving. This can bring forth important information about the particular problem the client is facing and can then enable structured discussion to take place. It allows room for clients to explore one particular problem in depth, while teaching them the process of problem-solving. The most valuable component of this approach is that it teaches the client how to slow down their reactions and to look objectively at a difficult situation. This widens their opportunities for finding solutions and increases their sense of personal efficacy.

Steps to Problem-solving

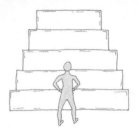

---

1. Define the problem: It is really important that you define the problem as it is for *you*; not anyone else. Be specific and personal. Do not think about solutions yet, simply define the problem in terms of wants, needs and feelings first.

---

2. Brainstorm any possible solutions: Allow yourself to write down *any* possible solutions, no matter how silly they seem. Do not evaluate the possible solutions yet, be creative and broad-minded. This will stop you from overlooking possible solutions.

---

3. Evaluate the possible solutions:

Possible solution	Advantages	Disadvantages
Go through the brainstormed list of possible solutions and pick the top five. Write them in this column and imagine each solution being implemented. Think of the advantages and disadvantages of each possible solution and write these in the next two columns. When you have done this, examine each solution and evaluate which has the most advantages and the least disadvantages.		

---

4. Select a solution and plan how to implement it: Select a solution and think about how you could implement it. Think about when and how you would put it into action, what resources you would need and whether you would need any help. Set a time to implement it.

---

5. Implement the plan and evaluate its success: Put the plan into action and evaluate how successful it was so that you can learn from it for next time. If it was not successful, go back to the list of brainstormed options and select another. Plan how to implement this option and review how it went afterwards.

Problem-solving

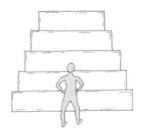

1. **Define the problem:**

2. **Brainstorm any possible solutions:**

3. **Evaluate the possible solutions:**

Possible solution	Advantages	Disadvantages

4. **Select a solution and plan how to implement it:**

5. **Implement the plan and evaluate its success:**

MAIN COURSE

SECTION 3 ANXIETY ISSUES

3.1 Psycho-education

This section contains psycho-educational handouts about anxiety, panic, worry, phobias and obsessive-compulsive disorder for the client to read in their own time or for the therapist to discuss with them during the course of therapy. Being educated about anxiety is very important in reducing the 'fear of the fear' that many anxiety sufferers describe.

What is Anxiety?

This sheet explains the normal physiological response of anxiety and its purpose in our survival. It then focuses on how anxiety can become unhelpful. This is a useful sheet for helping the client to understand the anxiety response and to heighten their awareness of their physical reactions.

What is a Panic Attack?

This is an educational sheet that explains the phenomenon of panic and its accompanying symptoms. It briefly lists some strategies for coping during a panic attack. This helps to demystify panic for sufferers, which can hopefully reduce some of the 'fear of the fear' associated with panic.

What is Worry?

The sheet explores the concept of worry, including some of the things that people worry about and the symptoms of worry and generalised anxiety. It also briefly lists some strategies for reducing worry and prompts the client to reflect on the things they worry about. This gives the therapist an opportunity to assess whether the client's level of worry is within the normal ranges or whether it is significantly impacting upon their life.

What is a Phobia?

In this handout, the two major types of phobias are discussed, including specific phobia and social phobia. It may be useful for a client suffering from a phobia to see that these are relatively common problems that respond well to treatment.

What is OCD?

This is an information sheet that outlines the major symptoms of obsessive-compulsive disorder (OCD). It provides a preliminary introduction into the complexities of OCD and lists some examples of obsessive thoughts and their accompanying compulsive behaviours. It briefly explains the maintaining factors of OCD, and its treatment.

What is Anxiety?

Anxiety is the name used to describe all the feelings and symptoms a person experiences when they feel that they are in danger. The feelings of caution, alarm, fear, terror, and panic are all part of anxiety.

Anxiety is our body's way of preparing and protecting us from danger. It is a physical response that is triggered firstly by our PERCEPTION of a THREAT in our environment. When we perceive something as dangerous (whether or not it is life-threatening) our body prepares us to FIGHT or FLIGHT for our survival. This is called the **fight/flight** response.

SOMETHING IN OUR ENVIRONMENT ⟶ WE *PERCEIVE* IT AS THREATENING ⟶ FIGHT/FLIGHT RESPONSE

The fight/flight response is **automatic** and sets about a range of changes in your body with the aim of helping you to fight or to run for your safety.

- **Breathing speeds up** to increase the amount of oxygen available for the muscles.

- **Heart rate and blood pressure increase** to distribute the oxygen and nutrients to the major muscles. Blood is diverted to the large muscles for this purpose and away from the organs, digestive system and the skin. This is why you feel sick and go pale when anxious.

- **Muscles tense**, preparing you for action.

- **Sweating increases** to keep your body cool should you start to engage in fight or flight.

- **Digestion** and other non-essential functions are temporarily put on hold until the danger passes. This can lead to nausea and diarrhoea.

- **The mind becomes preoccupied** with the threat and the danger and is not able to reason and concentrate as it normally would.

What is Anxiety? *cont.*

All of these symptoms serve a crucial function when you are faced with a life-threatening situation. However, your body will react in the **same way** whether you are **actually** faced with a serious danger or whether you simply PERCEIVE a situation as dangerous.

When you perceive a situation as dangerous, your body cannot tell whether that situation is life-threatening or not. **It will react in the same way regardless**. When a person's fight/flight response is repeatedly triggered over things that other people do not find threatening, it can impair their functioning and their happiness. This is when anxiety becomes a problem.

What is a Panic Attack?

A panic attack is the sudden onset of extreme anxiety. It can happen in different situations in which the person perceives there to be threat, but can sometimes even happen unexpectedly.

In panic attacks, the person will experience a lightning-fast increase in their anxiety. Panic attacks are frightening mainly due to their intensity and unpredictability, but are typically short-lived. Most people who experience panic are very fearful of having another attack and will avoid any situation in which they think they might panic. Unfortunately, this sets up a 'fear of the fear' within the person and prevents them from overcoming their panic.

Symptoms of a panic attack

The symptoms of a panic attack tend to peak within a ten-minute period of time and include some of the following:

- accelerated heart rate, pounding heart

- sweating

- trembling or shaking

- feelings of shortness of breath, smothering or suffocation

- sensation of choking or having a tight throat (lump in the throat)

- chest pain or discomfort

- feeling nauseous or experiencing abdominal pain

- dizziness, unsteadiness, feeling faint or light-headed

- feelings of unreality or of being detached from yourself

- fear of losing control or going crazy

What is a Panic Attack? *cont.*

- fear of dying

- numbness or tingling sensations

- chills or hot flushes.

What to do if you have a panic attack

To control panic, it is important to get help from a trained professional. Panic is highly treatable but without treatment, it can seriously limit a person's lifestyle and self-esteem.

First, learn to **recognise the warning signs** of an attack and respond quickly before it escalates. To do this, try to remove yourself from the situation and go to a quiet place where you can **breathe calmly and slowly**. Tell yourself that **you will survive this, it will pass and you can cope**.

Over-breathing (breathing too much air in rapid breaths – hyperventilation) is a major contributing factor in panic attacks. Therefore, learning to control and slow the breathing significantly helps to control panic. Eventually, it is important to be able to stay in the situation that triggers the attacks so that it does not limit your lifestyle, but this can be done in gradual steps with the help of a professional.

What is Worry?

Worry is when you focus on one or two things and think about them a lot of the time causing you to feel anxious and distressed.

Worrying causes anxious symptoms, such as:

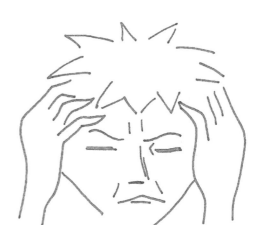

- nausea

- headaches

- tension

- agitation or restlessness

- sleeplessness

- fatigue

- difficulty concentrating

- irritability

- tearfulness.

Typically, people worry about things they can not control, such as:

- finances and money

- health

- loved ones (health/safety/happiness)

- work (pressure/relations/workload/colleagues/deadlines/satisfaction)

- life (future/past/mistakes).

What is Worry? *cont.*

Worrying for prolonged periods of time can affect your lifestyle and your health.

What to do to control worry

- Talk to someone about your worries.

- Make changes and take control in the areas that you can control.

- Accept the areas of your life that you cannot control.

- Schedule yourself half-an-hour a day as 'worry-time' and do not allow yourself to dwell on any issue outside of that time.

- Write your worries down on paper.

- Challenge your unrealistic worries with rational, realistic thoughts.

- Put plans into action to make changes in your life to reduce your worry.

- Set yourself goals to tackle the things that cause you worry.

What things do you worry about?

What is a Phobia?

A phobia is an extreme fear of a specific situation, environment or object. To be diagnosed as a phobia, the fear must be so extreme that it interferes with living a normal life. There are a lot of different types of phobias that fall into two groups.

1. **Specific phobia:** This is fear of specific situations or objects. The person feels intense anxiety if they are exposed to their feared situation or object and will avoid it any way they can. The level of anxiety they experience is far higher and more incapacitating than other people's reaction to the same situation or object. Some specific phobias include:

    *   storms

    *   heights

    *   water

    *   the dark

    *   animals – dogs, horses, birds etc.

    *   insects – spiders, cockroaches, moths etc.

    *   blood

    *   injury

    *   injections

    *   lifts/elevators

    *   bridges

    *   cars/buses/trains/aeroplanes

    *   crowds

    *   shopping centres

    *   enclosed spaces.

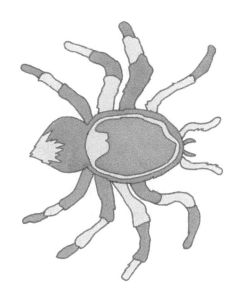

2. **Social phobia:** This is an intense fear of social situations where the person may be open to scrutiny by others. People suffering from social phobia are highly fearful of embarrassment or humiliation in these situations and try to avoid them at all cost. Some situations people with social phobia are fearful of are:

- public speaking

- meeting new people

- eating or drinking in front of others

- making small-talk

- writing in front of others

- entering a room full of people

- job interviews

- talking on the phone.

If you have a phobia that is interfering with your life, it is important to get help in overcoming it. By facing your fear in small steps, you can beat it. This will greatly increase your confidence and improve your life.

What is OCD?

Obsessive-compulsive disorder (OCD) is an anxiety disorder where people have a certain thought or image that enters their mind seemingly involuntarily and causes them significant anxiety and distress. This is called an **obsession** or, as it is sometimes termed, an intrusive thought.

People with OCD try to ignore or suppress these upsetting thoughts or images but find this impossible because they cause so much distress. These thoughts are more than everyday worries and OCD sufferers acknowledge that they are out of proportion, but have trouble setting them aside.

People suffering from OCD try to neutralise the anxiety caused by these thoughts by performing certain mental or behavioural acts, such as counting, washing, checking, or by performing other ritualistic behaviours. These behaviours, whether mental or behavioural, are called **compulsions**. The purpose of compulsions is to temporarily relieve the anxiety caused by the obsessions.

Some examples of obsessions and their possible accompanying compulsions are:

- *obsession:* intrusive worry about becoming sick and dying
  compulsion: excessive cleaning of hands and household surfaces

- *obsession:* intrusive fear of the house being broken into
  compulsion: repetitive checking of doors and windows

- *obsession:* intrusive fear that one could be a murderer/rapist
  compulsion: persistent avoidance of women, and self-punishment.

Obsessions and compulsions feed off each other and serve to maintain high levels of anxiety. This means that OCD sufferers have continually to find new and better ways of neutralising their anxiety. The catch is that the more they find ways to neutralise the anxiety caused by the obsessions, the worse the condition becomes. This is because they never prove their obsessive fear wrong.

Treatment involves understanding the links between obsessions and compulsions and breaking them by facing the anxiety evoked by the obsessions without the neutralising affect of the compulsions (therefore proving that the worst will not happen). Additionally, treatment requires challenging unhelpful patterns of thinking that maintain the anxious worries. Treatment is very difficult for OCD sufferers and they need intensive, specialist therapy and supportive helpers to bolster them through treatment.

3.2 Increasing awareness

This section contains activities to help increase the client's awareness of their anxiety and so prepare them for the application of the anxiety-reduction skills in the next section. It is important for the therapist to take the time to ensure that the client learns how to tune in to their anxiety in preparation for learning the skills to reduce it. Without the appropriate awareness, anxiety reduction skills are anchorless.

Monitoring my Anxiety

This sheet instructs the client to monitor their anxiety throughout the day, first by rating its severity out of 10, then by recording their symptoms, and finally by recording the events that were taking place at the time. This aims to increase the client's awareness of their environmental and internal triggers and to heighten their recognition of their subjective levels of anxiety.

Body Clues

In this exercise, the client records their physical symptoms of anxiety onto the picture. This could help the client to identify their symptoms in order to correctly interpret them and to catch their anxiety in its early stages. This is important for the client's understanding of the physical affects of anxiety, as well as for early identification of warning signs.

Early Warning System

This sheet encourages the client to explore the things that trigger their anxiety within themself and in their environment. It then helps them to identify their early warning sign that alerts them that they are becoming anxious. It is important that the therapist encourages the client to find their earliest possible warning sign in order for them to become accomplished in identifying their anxiety as early as possible. The earlier that anxiety is identified, the more effective the anxiety management strategies are. These insights are invaluable in reducing anxiety.

Monitoring my Anxiety

Throughout the day, keep an eye on your anxiety by monitoring it (0–10) and by recording your anxious symptoms and what was happening at the time.

TIME	RATE (0–10)	SYMPTOMS	WHAT WAS HAPPENING
Early morning			
Mid-morning			
Lunch			
Afternoon			
Evening			

Comments:

_____

_____

_____

Body Clues

Draw or write onto the diagram all of the feelings and symptoms you experience when you are feeling **ANXIOUS** or **SCARED**.

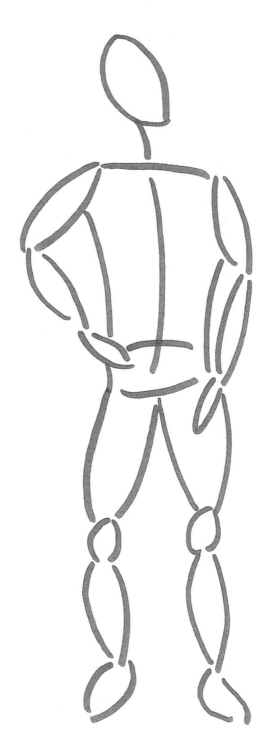

Early Warning System

To beat anxiety, it is important to have a good **early warning system**. This means that you need to know what things usually make you feel anxious (we call these **Triggers**), and you need to know straightaway when it is increasing (we call this your **Early warning sign**).

Triggers

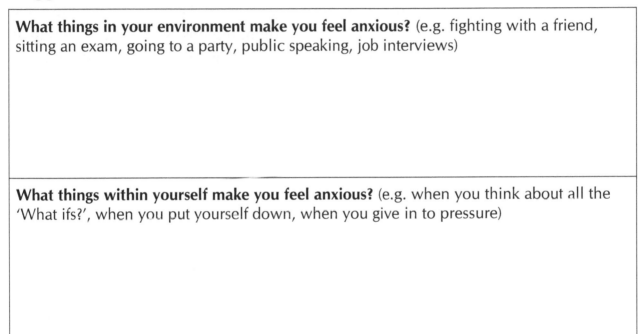

What things in your environment make you feel anxious? (e.g. fighting with a friend, sitting an exam, going to a party, public speaking, job interviews)

What things within yourself make you feel anxious? (e.g. when you think about all the 'What ifs?', when you put yourself down, when you give in to pressure)

Early warning sign

What physical feelings do you notice when you are starting to feel anxious (e.g. tense muscles, tight chest, heart pounding, sweating, sick in the stomach, want to cry, etc.)

3.3 Anxiety reduction strategies

In this section, the client is introduced to some proactive anxiety management techniques. Each technique has an accompanying worksheet or tip sheet for them to take away to aid in the generalisation of the skill into their life. These skills show the most success in clients who have good insight into their anxiety and are familiar with their triggers and waring signs. (See Section 3.2, Increasing awareness).

Slow Breathing

This sheet explains the role of over-breathing in the escalation of anxiety and panic and how to reduce the impact of the fight/flight response with slow breathing. It takes the client through the technique step by step. This is a valuable skill for clients that forms an important part of the treatment plan for anxiety. Therefore, this sheet might serve as a prompt for the client to understand and practise this skill. It is recommended that clients practise this skill several times a day so that it will be most effective when they are anxious.

Slow Motion

This is a brief technique that can be used to decrease the client's level of anxiety in the moment. It is not designed to solve the problem that is leading to their anxiety, it simply aims to help them manage at the time and reduce their levels of anxiety. It aims to improve the client's coping ability and confidence, and so equip them for further exploration of their anxiety.

Slow Motion is most effective if the therapist practises the skill with the client in session, using real life examples, and gives them a card with the points of the skill on it to trigger their recall. The sheet has three 'slow motion' cards on it, which the therapist can copy onto coloured card, and perhaps laminate, for distribution to their clients.

Relaxation

In this exercise the client is encouraged to reflect upon the amount of relaxation they have in their day-to-day life. For this exercise, relaxation is considered to be any form of activity that gives the client positive benefits, such as clearing the mind, time out, rest, play, recreation, release, etc. This allows the therapist to gain insight into the client's ability to take time for relaxation and their current situation.

Progressive Muscular Relaxation Script

This is a script that the therapist could read out, accompanied by music, in session to train the client in an active relaxation technique. It could also be given to the client to read for a homework task so that they understand how to talk themselves through this technique. The client could read this script out loud and record it onto a tape for themselves to use on a regular basis.

Passive Relaxation Script

This is similar to the above script, but this is a passive relaxation exercise that depicts a relaxing scene for the client to focus on while relaxing individual muscle groups. This simply demonstrates the technique and could be substituted for any relaxing scene that helps the client to relax. As with the above script, the therapist could read out the script in session or instruct the client to read it out loud, recording their voice onto a tape that they can use as required.

Slow Breathing

This is a very powerful breathing technique that reduces the symptoms of anxiety and helps you to think more clearly and to cope better when you feel anxious or stressed.

What does breathing have to do with ANXIETY and STRESS?

One of the first signals you give your body when faced with a threat is through your breathing. We all start to breathe more rapidly and shallowly when anxious or stressed and this sends a clear alarm signal to your body. This intensifies the **fight/flight** response.

Breathing rapidly when stressed can cause your levels of oxygen and carbon dioxide to become unbalanced, leaving you feeling light-headed and dizzy. This in turn can make you feel even more anxious, which sets up a vicious cycle of breathing and anxiety.

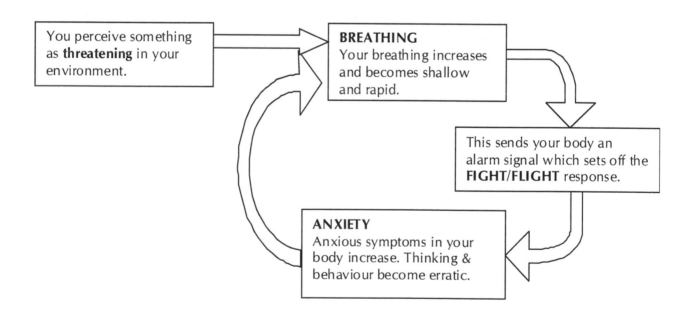

To reduce your anxiety, it is important to send your body a calm signal through your breathing. Instead of breathing rapidly and shallowly with your chest rising and falling, you need to breathe slowly and calmly so that your abdomen rises and falls in a smooth, slow rhythm.

How do you do 'slow breathing'?

First, you need to become aware of your breathing, especially when it becomes too shallow and rapid. If you notice this happening you need to hold your breath for 10 seconds, then exhale while saying 'RELAX' to yourself. Then, shut your mouth and breathe through your nose, taking slow controlled breaths in and out counting 'IN-TWO-THREE-PAUSE-OUT-TWO-THREE' slower and slower (not deeper and deeper!). Concentrate on your abdomen rising and falling rather than your chest, and think calm, soothing thoughts like 'I can cope, I will be fine, this will pass.'

Slow Motion

---

1. Monitor and name the emotion (0–10).

2. Look for your early warning sign.

3. **SLOW DOWN AND BREATHE:** abdominal breathing – 10 slow breaths.

4. Think calmly: **WHAT** is causing you to feel this way?

   WHY is this upsetting you? What can you

   DO to cope and reduce your feelings?

---

1. Monitor and name the emotion (0–10).

2. Look for your early warning sign.

3. **SLOW DOWN AND BREATHE:** abdominal breathing – 10 slow breaths.

4. Think calmly: **WHAT** is causing you to feel this way?

   WHY is this upsetting you? What can you

   DO to cope and reduce your feelings?

---

1. Monitor and name the emotion (0–10).

2. Look for your early warning sign.

3. **SLOW DOWN AND BREATHE:** abdominal breathing – 10 slow breaths.

4. Think calmly: **WHAT** is causing you to feel this way?

   WHY is this upsetting you? What can you

   DO to cope and reduce your feelings?

Relaxation

It is important for us all to relax. Relaxation allows our bodies to recharge and our minds to rest. This is very important for our general wellbeing and for our satisfaction with life.

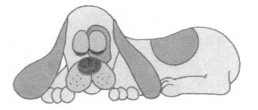

What do you do to relax?

Do you think you need to have more relaxation in your life? Why?

List some relaxing activities that you would like to do more of:

Set yourself a goal of increasing the amount of relaxation in your life.

My goal: _____

What would you need to do to make that happen?

Progressive Muscular Relaxation Script

Start by sitting or lying in a comfortable position where your head is supported and your feet and legs are uncrossed.

Begin by focusing your attention on your breathing. Make it smooth, slow and calm. Watch each breath as it slides in and washes out. Your breathing is effortless. It requires no tension, no worry and no interference. Breathe in slowly, pause, and then release the breath and along with it, any tension in your body. Pause before your next breath in, relishing the quiet that comes in that space where one breath leaves and another arrives. Extend that pause longer... and longer... with each breath.

Sink into your relaxation so that you feel and pay attention to every surface that touches your body. The fabric of your clothes lightly cocooning your body. The air passing over your skin, soothing you and smoothing away tension. You are so heavy that your body could continue sinking far, far beyond the chair or the floor that supports you.

Now take your attention to your feet. Tighten all the muscles in your feet by scrunching your toes. Hold that tension... Leave the rest of your body relaxed... HOLD...and release. Feel the warmth of relaxation return to your feet, enjoy that feeling. Now tighten your feet once more...HOLD...HOLD...and release. Revel in the relaxation of your feet. Let them become soft and pliable once more.

Now take your attention to your legs. Tense your calves and thighs...HOLD that tension...Harder...HOLD...and release. Let your legs become flooded with the warmth of relaxation. Let that feeling nourish the weary muscles. Enjoy that feeling. Now repeat the tension in your legs...HOLD...HOLD...and release. Feel the difference between cold, harsh, tension and warm, soothing relaxation. Let all of the tension wash away through your toes with each outward breath.

Now take your attention to your stomach, chest and back. Tense your whole torso by scrunching your stomach and collapsing your chest in on itself. HOLD that tension...HOLD...tighter...and release. Take a deep breath in, filling your whole chest cavity...HOLD...and sigh it out, releasing all pent-up tension and resistance. Feel the warmth of relaxation filling every part of your torso and trickling up your back. Spreading throughout your whole torso. Now repeat the tension...HOLD...HOLD...and release. Sigh the next breath out and enjoy the feeling of total relaxation. Let the tension flow out through your legs and feet, leaving only the tranquil, trickling feeling of relaxation.

Now take your attention to your arms and hands. Tense all the muscles of your hands and arms, making them rigid and tight...HOLD...HOLD...and release. Let them become soft and unyielding. Let them sink into the surface that supports them, feel them slightly disconnected from your body. Now repeat the tension...HOLD...HOLD... and release. Let the tension flow out through your fingertips.

Now turn your attention to your face and neck. Tense the muscles of your face and neck by scrunching up your face, clenching your jaw, and making your neck tight and stiff. HOLD...HOLD...and release. Take away all the tension of the day and let your face and neck become smooth, soft and relaxed. Let the relaxation melt into your face and neck. Spreading like the warmth of the sun, smoothing your brow, releasing your jaw and softening your neck. Now tighten your face and neck once more...HOLD...HOLD...and release.

Let the feeling of total relaxation spread from your face, down your neck...into your shoulders...down your arms...through your hands...filling all of your torso...and flowing down each of your legs...and pooling in your feet. With each breath in, breathe more relaxation into your body, and with each breath out, release more tension. Sinking deeper and deeper into your total relaxation. Enjoy that feeling for a few moments.

Now turn your attention to the room that you are in and the noises around you. Slowly start to stretch and move your body, and when you are ready, open your eyes and sit up, feeling refreshed and ready to deal with the next challenge you will face.

Passive Relaxation Script

Start by sitting or lying in a comfortable position where your head is supported and your feet and legs are uncrossed.

Begin by focusing your attention on your breathing. Make it smooth, slow and calm. Quiet your mind by concentrating on each and every breath. Your breath is like a tide, washing gently and smoothly in and quietly slipping back out. Take a deep breath in and hold it...then sigh the breath out, releasing tension, worry and tightness in your body. Your breathing is effortless. It soothes every corner of your body with its calming and life-giving presence. Allow your breathing to become slower and slower as you relax more and more.

Now bring your attention to your body. Begin to scan your body with your mind's eye, looking for any tension and releasing it. Sink into your relaxation so that you feel and pay attention to every surface that touches your body. The fabric of your clothes lightly touching your body. The air passing over your skin, soothing you and smoothing away tension. You are so heavy that your body could continue sinking far, far beyond the surface that supports you.

If your thoughts drift off onto other topics, don't dwell on them, simply allow them in and out again without paying them much attention. Re-focus on your breathing and the feelings in your body, now is the time to quiet your mind and nourish your body.

Begin to imagine that you are sitting in the sun on a cool day, feeling the sun warm your face, soothing it and releasing tension from it. Let all the tension flow away with each outward breath. Think of all the tiny muscles around your eyes, mouth, forehead, tongue, jaw, and relax them. Let them become soft. RELAX... Let your face smooth out and become completely free from tension. RELAX...

The sun begins to warm your shoulders and neck. It is warm and soothing, comforting and drawing away tension, letting it flow from your shoulders and neck out with each outward breath. Becoming soft and relaxed; warm and free of tension. Now the sun warms your arms and hands as well, warm and relaxed, feeling soft and loose, all tension flowing out with the help of the sun's peaceful presence. All the muscles in your arms and hands are free of tension, no longer tight. No longer ready to move, to react or to follow your will. Your face, neck, shoulders, arms and hands are flooded with the warmth and nourishment of relaxation.

The sun now begins to warm your torso, releasing tension from your chest and stomach. Your breath flows in and out, completely free of any resistance. Your abdomen is gently rising and falling with each inward breath. Your whole torso is relaxed and soft, filling with the warmth of the sun and the comfort of relaxation. All tension is released with each outward breath, flowing smoothly away, leaving only tranquillity. The sun is warm on your back, soothing it and encouraging any tightness and tension to melt away from your muscles, leaving them soft and relaxed. No longer needing to support you, the muscles of your back are embraced by the warmth of relaxation.

Now the sun is warming and soothing your legs, beginning to warm your thighs and calves, loosening those muscles and leaving them soft and pliant. Tension all flowing out. Enjoy the feeling of complete relaxation, all resistance gone. Feel your legs heavy and lethargic, no longer supporting your weight or carrying you. Loose and relaxed.

The warmth continues down to your feet, melting away the tightness, leaving total softness, calmness and peace. The tension flowing out through your feet with each outward breath. Now your whole legs are relaxed, heavy and loose. All resistance gone, leaving only stillness and warmth in its place.

Feel your whole body relaxed, quiet and calm. Enjoy the feeling of relaxation from head to toe. Allow the feeling to wash over your whole body with each inward breath, leaving you completely and totally relaxed. Relish that feeling for a few moments now, sinking deeper still.

Now become aware of your surroundings again, start to wriggle your fingers and toes, open your eyes, have a stretch if you like, and remember to keep the feeling of relaxation in mind whenever you feel tense, stressed or anxious.

3.4 Cognitive behavioural strategies for anxiety

This section provides cognitive and behavioural strategies specifically for anxiety. These techniques aim to complement the CBT strategies already discussed in Section 2.3, Cognitive behavioural therapy.

Exposure Therapy

This is a psycho-educational sheet that provides a rationale for exposure therapy in reducing anxiety and its related avoidance. It describes graded exposure using a hierarchy, and how this can greatly help people to overcome their fears. This sheet helps the client to feel fully informed about treatment in order for them to give their consent and to feel motivated to apply themselves to therapy.

For clients to be willing to make themselves acutely uncomfortable, as they undoubtedly will with exposure therapy, they need to fully understand the rationale. This is where this sheet and good psycho-education about the mechanisms of anxiety is invaluable. (See Section 3.1, Psycho-education).

Anxiety Hierarchy

This sheet allows the therapist and the client to develop a hierarchy for graded exposure therapy. It guides the client to break their fear down into steps and to record their overall level of anxiety while exposing themselves to that situation. This helps to structure exposure therapy and helps the client to review their progress.

It is important that the therapist guides this process to make sure that the client has manageable steps, realistic expectations, and the appropriate anxiety reduction strategies in place before attempting exposure therapy. The sheet allows for eight trials of each step however, this is only a guide. More or less repetition of each step might be needed to attain a lowered level of anxiety in that particular situation before proceeding to the next step. This should be explained to clients so that they do not feel disappointed if they need more than eight repetitions, or if they feel overwhelmed by the task of completing eight repetitions unnecessarily.

Exposure Therapy

When you are afraid of something, you will do all you can to AVOID it! This makes you feel good in the short term, but unfortunately, in the long term your fear will actually grow. The reason for this is that you never get a chance to prove your fears wrong.

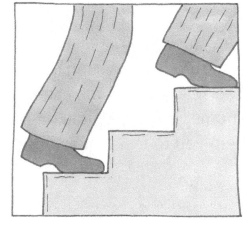

Therefore, in order to beat your fears, you need to face them! This is not easy. The most manageable way to do it is by breaking your fear down into small steps and tackling each step one by one. This means that your confidence grows with each step and your fear weakens.

How do I do it?

1. **Goal:** Be very clear about what your fear is and what your goal is. For example, a fear of dogs is rational, but if you were a vet you would need to overcome that fear to a higher level than someone who rarely comes into contact with dogs. Therefore, the goal for the vet might be to be able to treat and handle dogs with minimal anxiety. Another person's goal might be to be able to walk past houses with dogs in the yard with minimal anxiety. Each person has the same fear but a different goal in their individual lives.

2. **Steps:** Next, you need to break your fear down into small steps and to think about different situations where you will be exposed to varying levels of anxiety. Arrange these situations in order, from the easiest to the hardest, and give them a rating out of ten for how anxious you would be if confronted by that situation now.

3. **Start:** Start with the first step and rate your anxiety before, during and after your exposure to the situation. Stay in the situation long enough for your fear to decrease a little. Tell yourself positive thoughts and use slow breathing. Repeat that same step over and over until you can do it with minimal anxiety.

Exposure Therapy *cont.*

4. **Challenge:** Challenge yourself to move on to the next step after you feel comfortable (moderately) with the first step. As your confidence increases, keep moving up until you achieve your goal!

Tips

Have a support person to help motivate you and to stop you from avoiding. Give yourself rewards for each step. Make sure the progression from one step to another is gradual; you might need to break your steps down more as you go, to help you to feel that each step is attainable.

Anxiety Hierarchy

GOAL: _____

Your **expected** level of anxiety (0–10)	FEARED SITUATIONS	**Exposure 1** Rate overall level of anxiety	**Exposure 2** Rate overall level of anxiety	**Exposure 3** Rate overall level of anxiety	**Exposure 4** Rate overall level of anxiety	**Exposure 5** Rate overall level of anxiety	**Exposure 6** Rate overall level of anxiety	**Exposure 7** Rate overall level of anxiety	**Exposure 8** Rate overall level of anxiety

SECTION 4 DEPRESSIVE ISSUES

4.1 Psycho-education

These sheets are designed to give an introduction to the concept of depression and to increase the client's awareness of the effect that depression can have in their life. They provide opportunity for discussion during therapy and for later reading and digesting by the client.

These strategies will compliment worksheets from other sections of this book but are designed to target specific depression-related symptomatology. They are best used with clients whose primary difficulties derive from depression.

What is Depression?

This information sheet describes the symptoms of depression in detail and encourages the client to list their own symptoms. This can lead to open discussion about the impact of their depressive symptoms on their life and can provide important information about the client's needs for change. This can, therefore, guide the treatment plan.

Grief and Loss

This is an information sheet that aims to help clients to understand the process of grief and loss. It emphasises that grieving is an individual experience and that all people grieve in different ways. It is intended to validate the client's experience of grief and to encourage them to accept their own journey of healing.

What is Depression?

Depression is a mental illness where people feel intensely sad, down and hopeless. It completely interferes with their lives and affects every aspect of a person's thinking, feeling and interaction with others.

Symptoms of depression

- extremely depressed mood all day, for nearly every day for a prolonged period of time (at least two weeks)

- no interest in activities or pleasure

- negative, pessimistic and hopeless thinking patterns

- thoughts of death, suicidal thoughts, self-criticism and self-blame

- feelings of guilt, anger, anxiety and worthlessness

- difficulty concentrating, making decisions and managing stress

- sleep pattern changes – typically, people cannot get to sleep for hours, then finally drop off in the early hours, only to waken a few hours later to repeat the cycle again

- sleep disturbance leads to lethargy, lack of motivation and fatigue

- appetite changes – for some their appetite increases, which can lead to weight gain and its associated problems for body image and self-esteem. For others, their appetite reduces, leading to weight loss and low energy

- people suffering from depression often avoid social interaction and withdraw into isolation

- depressive symptoms stop a person from living a normal life. They interfere with family life, work life and social and recreational life.

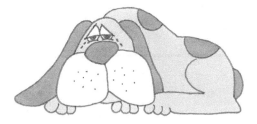

What is Depression? *cont.*

What are some of your symptoms of depression?

Grief and Loss

Each person's experience of grief and loss is individual to them. There is no set response that you 'should' have or any predictable order that you will follow in your grieving experience. However, most people will encounter some of these feelings, sometimes more than once.

DENIAL: disbelief, shock, and numbness. This is often because the mind sometimes needs to protect itself from the reality and pain of the loss.

ANGER: rage, recrimination, protest and hostility. These feelings can surface when the individual realises the loss but finds it hard to accept the injustice. Anger can be directed at the loved one, at yourself or at others.

DESPAIR: sadness, crying, hopelessness, and abandonment. These feelings can consume the bereaved, making it difficult to think of anything else.

GUILT: what if…? If only…? These feelings stem from feelings of responsibility, blame and wishful thinking that always accompany a loss.

CONFUSION: disorientation, lack of direction and bewilderment. Loss challenges your view of the world, changes your perspective and causes you to question yourself. Focus, concentration and decision-making are affected.

ACCEPTANCE: Gradually, you may be able to accept the reality of the loss and to find some hope for the future. By gathering meaning from the loss, you might also be able to start to set goals for your own life.

Hints for dealing with grief

- Give yourself permission to grieve in your own way.

- Don't bottle your feelings up – release them in healthy ways.

- Don't run away from the pain. The pain will lessen only by your facing it.

- Surround yourself with all that is familiar; people, places and surroundings.

- Don't put a time limit on your grief – it will be done when it is done.

- It is OK to have fun sometimes – this does not diminish your grief or mean that you don't care.

- Make small goals; be aware of your limitations.

- Try to find some meaning in the loss without diminishing its importance, e.g. parts of the loved one that live on in you, lessons they taught you, what they would want for your life.

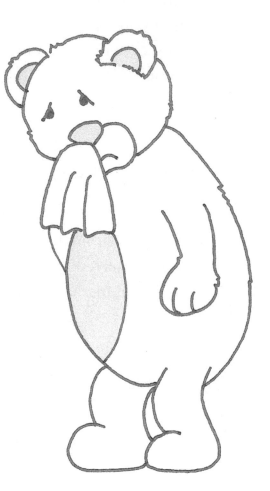

4.2 Behavioural strategies for depression

This section contains a monitoring sheet to assess the client's level of functioning, and activities to increase behavioural activation in clients suffering predominantly from depression. It also addresses some of the motivational issues that might prevent depressed clients from commencing or sticking to a behavioural activation program.

Activity Monitoring

This is a monitoring sheet for assessing a client's level of activity throughout a week. It enables the therapist to determine the impact of depressive symptoms on the client's functioning, as well as providing a baseline prior to behavioural activation. This can really emphasise the impact of depression for some clients, which can then serve as a strong motivation for getting back in control of their lives.

Pleasant Activities

This sheet provides a list of activities that can lift the mood of a depressed client. It provides an exhaustive list of options, as well as serving as a visual prompt for pleasant activities. Additionally, it might help the therapist and client to discuss the importance of pleasant events in the recovery from depression.

Increasing Activity Levels

This sheet explains the importance of pleasant activity in the treatment of depression and encourages the client to think of two activities they would like to do more of. The 'Pleasant Activities' list from the previous sheet might serve as a prompt for this. Once the client has selected two activities, they could then use a 'My Goal' sheet from Section 2.5, Goal-setting, to further plan this activity.

Barriers to Activity

This sheet lists some of the reasons why people put off or avoid activity. This enables the client to identify their personal barriers and to discuss them with the therapist so that they can be tackled individually.

Destructive Things I do when I am Down

This exercise explores the activities that clients might engage in when they are feeling depressed and which could have a negative impact on their mood and their life. With the use of this sheet, these activities are brought up for discussion with the therapist and more helpful activities can then be generated. This allows for open discussion about the possibility of self-harm or any other self-destructive coping strategies that the client might be employing.

Activity Monitoring

Name: _____   **Date:** _____

ACTIVITY	MONDAY	TUESDAY	WEDNESDAY	THURSDAY	FRIDAY	SATURDAY	SUNDAY
7am							
8am							
9am							
10am							
11am							
12pm							
1pm							
2pm							
3pm							
4pm							
5pm							
6pm							
7pm							
8pm							
9pm							

Pleasant Activities

Talking to a friend

Singing

Dancing

Listening to music

Collecting things

Going for a holiday

Setting goals

Relaxing

Having a long bath or shower

Swimming

Snorkelling

Patting your dog or cat

Watching the sun set

Being by the water

Listening to the sounds of nature

Going on a date

Jogging

Smiling

Calling a friend for a chat

Acknowledging what you have done well

Lying in the sun

Listening to others

Planning a career change

Laughing

Telling jokes

Reading

Watching TV

Exercise

Finishing something

Getting dressed up

Buying yourself something new

Spending time with friends

Going to the movies

Making something from scratch

Hugging

Listening to live music

Hobbies

Repairing something

Giving someone a gift

Ice-skating or rollerblading

Walking

Drawing or painting

Lying in a peaceful place

Arts and crafts

Kissing

Chocolate

Telling someone you love them

Doing absolutely nothing

Thinking about your own good qualities

Having breakfast in bed

Sleeping

Seeing a good movie

Doing something for someone else

Horseriding

Bushwalking

Surfing

Walking on the beach

Staying up all night

Eating your favourite meal

Meeting new people

Going camping

Arranging flowers

Diving into cool water

Praying

Getting together with your family

Cleaning

Sewing

Sightseeing

Going for a picnic

Being pampered

Photography

Fishing

Writing in a diary or journal

Acting/drama

Stargazing

Learning something new

Looking through photos

Lighting candles or incense

Getting a massage

Going skiing

Sleeping in

Gardening

Playing team sports

Driving

Flying a kite

Afternoon naps

Playing with a dog

Playing a musical instrument

Entertaining

Writing stories or poetry

Games with children

Going to the theatre

Bike riding

Exploring the internet

Cooking

Seeing live sport

Sailing

Being alone

Having a deep discussion

Meditating

Playing cards

Scrapbooking

Having coffee at a café

Going to museums or art galleries

Going windowshopping

Believing that 'I'm OK'

Increasing Activity Levels

One way to overcome depression is to increase your general activity levels by doing more things that you enjoy. The symptoms of depression, such as tiredness, lethargy, lack of motivation and loss of pleasure can make this very difficult, so set small goals to build up your level of activity gradually.

At first, you may not enjoy certain activities, but remember that at least you are taking an active step to beat depression. If you persevere, you will gradually start to enjoy it.

What are two things you would like to do more of?

1. _____

Why? _____

How can you start this? _____

_____

2. _____

Why? _____

How can you start this? _____

_____

Barriers to Activity

It won't make me
feel better.

It's too expensive.

I don't feel well
enough.

My back/feet/head
hurts.

I don't want to do
it by myself.

I have too
many other things
to do first.

I don't have the
time.

If I do something
for me I am selfish.

I don't have
enough energy.

Fear of failure.

I can't start.

There's no point
because I won't
stick to it.

It will only be
disappointing
anyway.

I have to look
after everyone
else first.

If I can't do it
perfectly I won't
do it at all!

I can't say NO!

Destructive Things I do when I am Down

List in the left column some of the things you do when you are feeling down that have a negative impact on your life. Record what that negative impact is and then, in the right column, list some more helpful activities you could do to help you to feel a bit better.

Destructive things I do	Impact they have	More helpful things I could do

4.3 Cognitive strategies for depression

This section aims to add to the material already discussed in the Therapy Basics section, specifically Section 2.3, Cognitive behavioural therapy. The techniques described here help to tailor cognitive therapy to the individual presenting predominantly with depressive issues.

The Role of Thinking in Depression

This is a monitoring sheet with a focus on depressed thoughts. It aims to help the client to become aware of the impact of their thinking on their mood, and to see that more severe, irrational cognitions lead to more intense feelings of sadness. This can then serve as evidence for changing unhelpful cognitions.

Positive Thinking Cue Cards

These cue cards are designed to be used following a 'Changing your Thinking' sheet (from page 74 in Section 2.3, Cognitive behavioural therapy). The aim of this exercise is for the client to write down some realistic, positive thoughts onto a cue card so that they can refer to them regularly. This aids in the learning of new patterns of thinking and serves as a reminder for the client of their new, more helpful ways of thinking.

Without Depression…

This sheet explores the possibility of life without depression and begins to build a new cognitive script. It allows discussion and re-authoring of the client's journey with depression and their future without it. This can greatly improve a client's motivation to tackle their issues and change negative patterns of thinking and behaviour.

The Role of Thinking in Depression

Throughout the day, monitor your level of depressed feelings and rate them out of 10. Whenever your feelings are over 5, pay attention to what is happening and what you are thinking, and record it below.

What was happening	Rate 0–10	What you were thinking

What do you notice about your thoughts? Are there any patterns? _____

_____

_____

_____

_____

_____

Positive Thinking Cue Cards

Positive thoughts

1. _____

   _____

2: _____

   _____

3. _____

   _____

4. _____

   _____

Positive thoughts

1. _____

   _____

2: _____

   _____

3. _____

   _____

4. _____

   _____

Positive thoughts

1. _____

   _____

2: _____

   _____

3. _____

   _____

4. _____

   _____

Positive thoughts

1. _____

   _____

2: _____

   _____

3. _____

   _____

4. _____

   _____

Without Depression…

Without depression, my life will be: _____

_____

_____

Without depression, I will be able to: _____

_____

_____

Without depression, I will feel: _____

_____

_____

Without depression others will: _____

_____

_____

Without depression, I will start to: _____

_____

_____

Without depression, the real me: _____

_____

_____

5 ANGER ISSUES

5.1 Psycho-education

The sheets and activities in this section explore the concept of anger as an emotion and investigate some of the common causes of anger. All of these exercises aim to help the client to understand and label their experience of anger. Some clients have difficulty identifying their anger or accepting that they have angry feelings. For this reason, this section aims to look at the positives and negatives of anger rather than simply seeing it as a negative experience.

What is Anger to Me?

This is a psycho-educational and self-exploratory sheet that encourages the client to explore the things that make them feel angry and the symptoms they experience when angry. It concludes by discussing the concept of anger as an emotion with a view to increasing the client's insight into their perception of their world and their expectations. This may allow the therapist to validate the client's realistic expectations and their appropriate anger and to gently challenge some of the client's unrealistic expectations that could be inflaming or maintaining their anger.

Types of Anger

This is an educational sheet that describes some of the different ways that people express and deal with their anger. This aims to familiarise clients with the many forms of anger and to help increase their insight into their own methods of expressing their anger.

Anger...What's Behind it?

This sheet encourages the client to look beyond their anger and to examine the underlying or primary emotions that are contributing to the development of their anger. It opens up discussion about the causes of anger and helps the client and therapist to explore the deeper issues involved. This can help clients to view anger as a secondary reaction that signals the existence of an underlying issue.

Sometimes, this can make anger less threatening or unpalatable for clients who struggle to allow themselves to feel angry, because they can view it as a useful sign to look deeper. For clients who are familiar with and accepting of their anger, this discussion can prompt them to look beyond the surface-level emotion and uncover the motivations and causes for their anger.

What is Anger to Me?

What does anger mean to you?

How do you know when you are feeling angry? What do you feel and do?

What sorts of things make you feel angry? Why?

Anger is a normal emotional response that lets you know that your expectations have not been met. When something in your life does not go as you expected it to, it is normal to have a reaction to that.

Think about some of the things that make you angry and see if there is a difference between what you expected to happen and what did happen...

Are your expectations always reasonable and appropriate?

Can you adjust your expectations to help your anger to decrease? How?

Types of Anger

All people express anger in their own way. Anger can take many forms, below are some for the many ways that anger can be experienced.

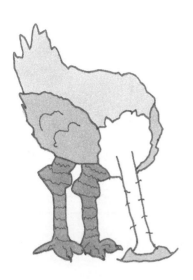

HEAD IN THE SAND

Some people find anger frightening or unacceptable. They shy away from acknowledging or expressing angry feelings and instead convince themselves that they are *not angry*. The problem with this coping mechanism is that they do not release and express their feelings, which can lead to a build-up of resentment and unhappiness.

> *'I'm fine, I'm not angry at all.'*
> *'I don't mind.'*

RETREATING TO THE CAVE

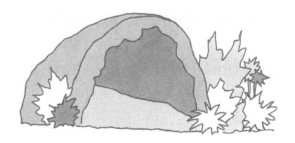

Other people find anger so difficult to deal with that they do all that they can to *avoid* it. They try to hide in their 'cave' whenever they feel angry or whenever people around them are angry. Unfortunately, this means that they do not learn to manage their anger or other people's anger.

> *'I can't deal with this right now.'*
> *'Let's talk about something else and just get along.'*
> *'I suddenly realised that I forgot to buy milk.'*

BOTTLERS

Some people find it very hard and very frightening to express their angry feelings, so they push them away and *hold onto* them deep inside. This can be because they fear conflict or because they don't think they have a right to feel angry. Either way, bottling up angry feelings is like a ticking bomb that can lead to big explosions over little things down the track.

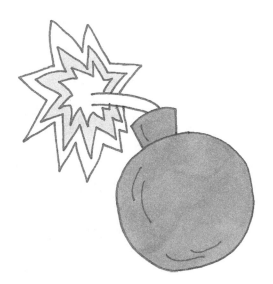

'I can't say anything because it will cause a fight.'

'It's not that bad.'

'Nothing will change.'

EXPLODERS

Some people yell and scream and 'blow off steam' when they are angry. They explode, lashing out at others either verbally or physically. This can provide a satisfying *release* for them in the short term, but can have devastating consequences in the long term for themselves and their relationships.

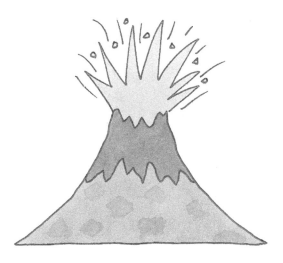

'You stupid #@$%!'

'I'm right; everyone else is in the wrong and deserves to pay!'

Anger... What's behind it?

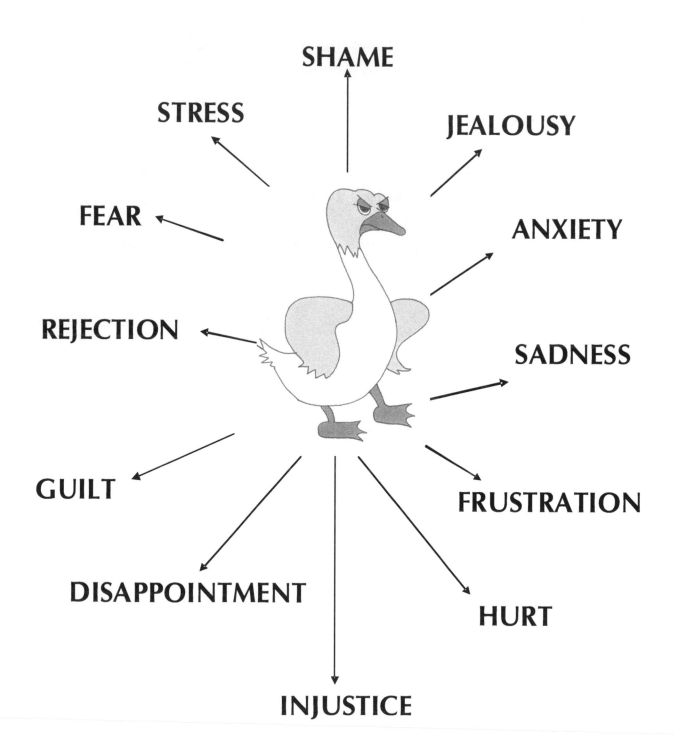

SHAME

STRESS

JEALOUSY

FEAR

ANXIETY

REJECTION

SADNESS

GUILT

FRUSTRATION

DISAPPOINTMENT

HURT

INJUSTICE

5.2 Motivation for managing anger

The following sheets help the client and therapist to further explore anger, particularly relating to the impact that anger has on the client's life. The client is non-judgementally encouraged to reflect upon the situations that make them angry and their reactions to these stressors. This allows for discussion about the advantages and disadvantages of anger for them, and for the therapist to assess the client's level of motivation to change.

Monitoring and Exploring Anger

This sheet guides the client to think about the situations in which they become angry and why. It asks them to reflect upon the thoughts they have when angry and the actions they usually take. This then allows for discussion about the usefulness and appropriateness of their responses to anger.

Advantages and Disadvantages of Anger

In this exercise, the client is asked to contemplate their attachment to their anger and its associated behaviours by weighing up the advantages and disadvantages of having anger in their life. This is especially useful for clients who are somewhat 'stuck' by their anger and seem unable to let it go despite acknowledging its negative consequences in their life.

It is important that the therapist is completely non-judgemental throughout this process and allows the client to come to whatever conclusion they are ready to come to in relation to their anger. Only if the client decides for themselves that anger has too many disadvantages for it to be a productive part of their life will they be motivated to align with the therapist to tackle it. This serves as a useful gauge for the therapist to determine a client's level of motivation to work on their anger.

What I do with my Anger

This sheet aims to help clients to explore their particular method of managing their anger. It is especially useful for clients who bottle or deny their anger. It asks them what they would *like* to do (but never do) when they are angry; and to investigate why there is a difference between what they want to do and actually do with their anger. Some common roadblocks to releasing anger are then listed for the client to reflect on and to discuss with their therapist.

Monitoring and Exploring Anger

Anytime you feel angry (no matter how much or how little), record what happened in the table below:

What happened? Rate your anger (0–10)	Why did this make you feel angry?	What thoughts went through your mind?	What did you do (good or bad)?	Did these actions make you feel better or worse?

Advantages and Disadvantages of Anger

Think about anger in your life... What are the good things about it and the bad things about it?

ADVANTAGES	DISADVANTAGES

Considering these things, is anger a helpful or unhelpful part of your life?

What I do with my Anger...

What I really want to do but don't do when I feel angry is:

-
-
-
-

What I actually do when I feel angry is:

-
-
-
-

Why is there a difference between what you would like to do and what you actually do when you are angry?

Read through this list of roadblocks to releasing anger and tick those that apply to you:

- fear of hurting others (emotionally or physically)
- fear of ruining relationships
- fear of conflict
- feeling that anger is uncomfortable and unpleasant

- believing that you 'shouldn't' be angry

- worry that you will be judged for being angry

- feeling that you might lose control if you release your anger

- believing that anger is a weakness

- feeling that you should be able to 'deal with it' and stay calm

- believing that 'nice' people don't get angry

- fear that others will reject you if you are angry

- fear of the feeling of being angry – scary, unattractive, negative.

5.3 Anger management

The sheets in this section provide useful and practical strategies for managing anger in both the short and long term. They include strategies for immediate reduction of anger, as well as strategies for challenging the triggers and cognitions behind angry emotions.

Dealing with your Anger

This is an information sheet that provides the client with a list of strategies for reducing anger in the short and long term. This may be useful as a discussion tool during therapy or as an information sheet for the client to take home. The main focus is on empowering the client to respond to their anger in healthy rather than unhealthy ways, and to make changes in their life and in their relationships to reduce the frequency of triggers for their anger.

Anger Management

In this exercise, the client is made aware of the role of thinking in the escalation of anger and aggression. Links are made between thoughts, feelings and behaviours in order to highlight the importance of attuning to angry thoughts and challenging them to reduce anger.

Personal Anger Management Plan

This sheet summarises for the client their personal approach to anger management. It asks them to list their triggers, warning signs, and 'hot' thoughts that escalate their anger. It then asks them to list their chosen strategies for managing their anger. This serves as a quick reference for regular use by the client.

Dealing with your Anger

Anger can be a very difficult emotion to deal with. Here are some tips to help you to manage your anger appropriately.

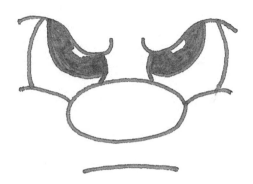

BEFORE YOU GET ANGRY...

1. Recognise that anger is a normal reaction, that it can be healthy and productive.

2. Remember that you are responsible for your feelings and your actions.

3. Anger and aggression are not the same thing. Anger is a normal and healthy emotion. Anger can become aggression if it is channelled into inappropriate and harmful acts towards others.

4. Become familiar with the things that trigger your feelings of anger and try to make changes in your life to reduce them.

5. Know your personal warning signs that you are becoming angry.

6. Learn to recognise the things that you do when angry that are not healthy for you.

7. Develop coping strategies to help you to reduce the frequency of your anger. For example, get more relaxation, communicate openly with your family and friends about the things that bother you, take more time for things you enjoy.

8. Make changes spontaneously. As soon as something happens that makes you feel the early warning signs of anger, speak up, assertively and respectfully.

Dealing with your Anger *cont.*

WHEN YOU GET ANGRY...

1. Catch it early and do something *immediately* to prevent it from escalating.

2. Walk away, be alone, take five long, slow deep breaths counting backwards from five.

3. Think about whether this situation is one that you need to work out with the other person or one that you need to resolve within yourself.

4. Tell the other person that you need time to think things through and that you want to talk more about this in half-an-hour. It is very important that the other person understands that you need space to gather your thoughts in order to prevent the escalation of your anger.

5. Go away and think about WHAT exactly upset you and WHY, think about what you need to SAY to the other person involved that will help a *resolution* to be found (not to score points!).

Managing Anger

Anger is not always easy to manage, mainly due to its intensity and the behaviours we associate with anger (aggressive behaviours such as yelling, screaming, swearing, hitting, throwing things, etc.). If you recognise that anger can be a problem in your life, pay special attention to the things you tell yourself when you are angry BEFORE you act on your anger.

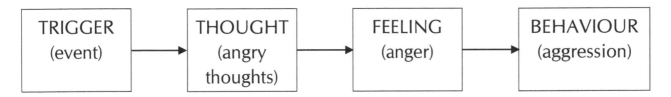

| TRIGGER (event) | → | THOUGHT (angry thoughts) | → | FEELING (anger) | → | BEHAVIOUR (aggression) |

By changing the way you think when you are angry, you can change the way you feel. This, in turn, can reduce aggressive behaviours and their related negative consequences.

Angry thoughts

Learn to identify the thoughts that fuel your anger and to challenge them. Make them into more helpful thoughts.

Think of the last time you felt angry.

What happened?

_____

_____

_____

What thoughts went through your mind that fuelled your anger?

_____

_____

_____

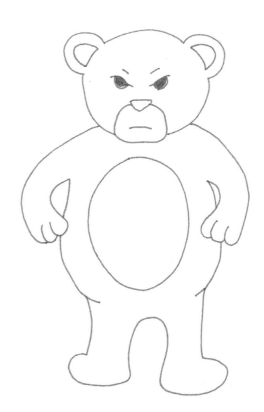

Helpful thoughts

Ask yourself the following questions to help challenge your angry thoughts:

Is this really worth it?

- Will it matter in a week's time?

- What do you want to gain from this situation? Is this likely?

- What are the feelings behind my anger?

- What needs to happen for me to feel better about this?

- What can I do to resolve this?

Now turn each angry thought into a more helpful thought:

_____

_____

_____

_____

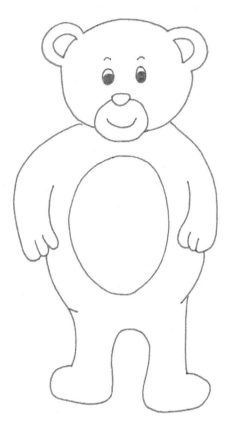

Personal Anger Management Plan

Anger is a problem for me when: _____

_____

_____

_____

The **triggers** for my anger are: _____

_____

_____

_____

My personal **early warning** that I am getting angry is: _____

_____

_____

_____

Steps I can take to be READY to catch my anger are: _____

_____

_____

_____

Personal Anger Management Plan *cont.*

In order to STEADY my anger, things I can tell myself are:

_____

_____

_____

Things I can do to prevent myself from doing something I will later regret are: _

_____

_____

_____

Why this is worth doing: _____

_____

_____

_____

SECTION 6 COMMUNICATION SKILLS

6.1 Communication skills

Many issues that cause unhappiness stem from poor communication. Learning to communicate better with others and to express one's own feelings and needs is vital to emotional wellbeing. This section contains worksheets, tip sheets and exercises to encourage clients to explore and improve their relationships with others through communication.

Communication

This sheet explains the process of communication with a focus on the verbal and nonverbal components and how the message can be affected by many factors in the communication process. The aim of this information sheet is to outline how complicated communication can be, so that clients can begin to gain a deeper understanding of their own and others' messages.

Friendships

This is a simple sheet that opens up discussion about friendships in the client's life. This is especially useful to work through with clients who have expressed a desire to have more friends or who have conveyed a reluctance to pursue friendships as a result of their own fears.

Listening

This tip sheet outlines the important ingredients required to be a good listener. This is a useful tool for training clients in the art of listening and could be used to prompt them through the steps while role-playing with the therapist, or as a homework reading task.

People in my Life

This exercise asks the client to reflect upon the interpersonal relationships they have in their life and the relative closeness of those relationships. This helps the therapist to ascertain the client's level of social support, and the client to consider their satisfaction with their interpersonal relationships and social supports. It raises the concept of intimacy and closeness to people based on authentic sharing of feelings. This might lead to discussion about sharing of feelings and opinions with others and barriers to intimacy in interpersonal relationships.

Relationships

This sheet uses the analogy of a garden to discuss the concept of relationships and their maintenance. It aims to make the client think about how much they nurture themselves while in a relationship (either a romantic relationship or a friendship). It also looks at how much each party puts into the relationship and what happens when there is an imbalance in this area. This may be a useful analogy for encouraging clients to reflect upon imbalances in their relationships and to stress the importance of nurturing themselves while in a relationship.

Early Relationship Lessons

This exercise aims to develop insight into the client's approach to social and emotional relationships as learned in their family of origin. This is especially useful for opening up discussion about early learning experiences in the family and interpersonal interactions in the client's family home. This may uncover systems of beliefs about relationships, assertiveness and conflict, based on early learning experiences.

Communication Roadblocks

This sheet briefly lists some of the roadblocks that can halt communication in relationships. It might be a constructive tool for encouraging clients to objectively examine some of the traps they fall into when communicating with others (especially when emotional). This links in with the previous sheet about early learning experiences from the family of origin, and might provide useful material for discussion about communication patterns in the client's life.

Communication

Communicating with another is a complicated process! It involves sending and receiving a message. However, many factors influence how that message is sent and how it is received.

THE ENVIRONMENT

The environment affects how well a message is sent and recieved. Things such as distractions, other people, noise, heat, cold, and time constraints all play a role.

YOU

Something you want to communicate starts here as a thought.

How you communicate it depends on:

- Your mood
- Past experiences
- Your confidence
- Your attitides and expectations
- How well you have thought through your message
- How you convey it
- Much more!

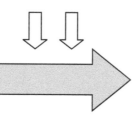

THE MESSAGE

35% of the message is verbal:

the words that are used, how those words are used (spoken, written, sung, in person, over the phone), clarity of the message.

65% of the message is non-verbal: tone of voice, volume, inflection, body language, behaviour, facial emphasis, gestures, emphasis on particular words, emotion level.

THE OTHER PERSON

Perceives the message and responds based on:

- Their level of attention and hearing
- The effort of their listening
- Their level of emotionality
- Their openness to the message
- Their own past experiences and expectations
- Their understanding
- Much more!

We place far more emphasis on the nonverbal channel of communication and if there is a discrepancy between verbal and nonverbal, we will always believe the nonverbal (actions speak louder than words). An example of this is, if someone said to you, 'I like you' but did not make eye-contact with you and walked away while speaking, you would not put much faith in their liking for you. However, if they said these same words while looking at you, smiling and touching you on the arm, you would be much more inclined to believe them.

Therefore, to communicate well, you need to think about the message you want to send and make sure that your verbal and nonverbal communication channels are in line and that you think about how the message will be received by the other.

Friendships

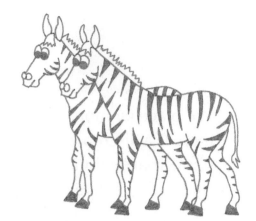

Describe your ideal friend:

In what ways are you a good friend?

What have your experiences been with friends in the past?

What would you like to gain from making a new friend?

What fears do you have about making a new friend?

Listening

1. **Want to listen!** Almost all problems can be resolved by listening to the other person in an open and respectful way. Even the most upset and irrational person will calm down and become reasonable if they are listened to. Listening makes people feel validated and understood.

2. **Give the other person your complete attention.** This might mean that you have to stop what you are doing or schedule in a time to talk when you can give them your full attention.

3. **Listen in a non-judgemental frame of mind.** Be open to their concerns and try to put yourself in their position. Even if you don't agree with their argument, they have the right to express it.

4. **Do not interrupt them.** Let them completely finish what it is that they have to say. Interruptions can be interpreted as argument by the speaker and will leave them feeling invalidated. The only time interruption is welcome is when the other person is being applauded. Do this generously but briefly!

5. **Encourage them through your body language** by giving them eye-contact, leaning forward, looking interested and nodding. Use minimal encouragers like 'oh', 'really' and 'go on' to let them know that you are with them and that you are giving them your complete attention.

6. **Where appropriate, reflect their feelings** in your body language and facial expression and by saying things like, for example, 'That sounds very upsetting' or 'You seem very hurt by that'. This shows them that you are identifying with their feelings and that you understand where they are coming from.

Listening *cont.*

7. **When they have finished or pause, paraphrase** (summarise in your own words) what they have said to clarify that you understand and to show the other that you are concerned, interested and trying to work with them.

8. **Ask questions** when you don't understand, when you need to clarify or when you want the other person to think about their feelings. This will help them to solve their problem themselves. For instance, 'What upsets you the most about this?' or 'What do you see as a possible solution?'

Do you think you are a good listener? What do you do well and what could you improve upon?

_____

_____

_____

_____

_____

People in my Life

Write into the diagram all of the people who play a role in your life:

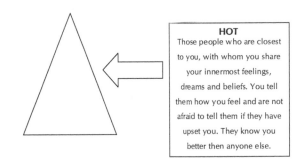

HOT
Those people who are closest to you, with whom you share your innermost feelings, dreams and beliefs. You tell them how you feel and are not afraid to tell them if they have upset you. They know you better then anyone else.

WARM

Those people who you are close to, can be yourself with and share your feelings with, but who might not know all there is to know about you. Close friends.

LUKEWARM

Those people with whom you can share a laugh and offer an opinion but you do not feel very close to. These are people who you could become closer to in time.

COOL

Those people with whom you interact but share nothing of yourself.

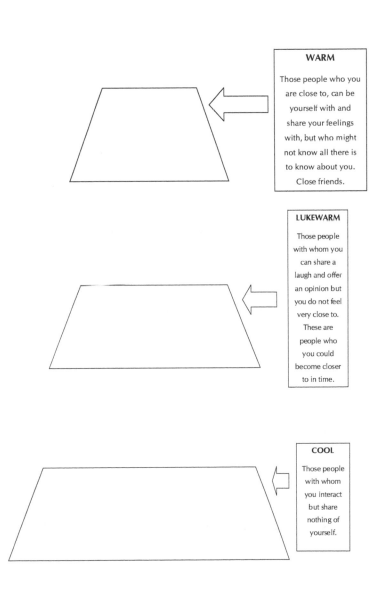

Relationships

A relationship is like a garden that needs watering and feeding by both parties in order to flourish. Each individual in the relationship is responsible for themselves (their own garden) and the relationship (the joint garden).

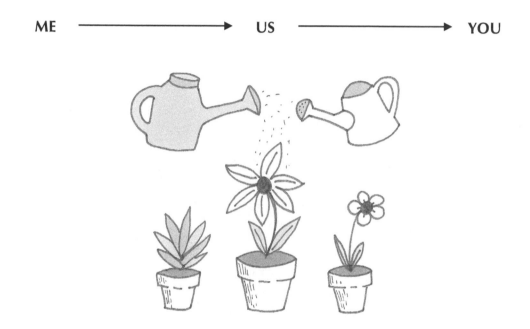

ME ⟶ US ⟶ YOU

In times of trouble for one person, the other may have to help to water their garden as well as their own. This is sustainable for short periods of time, but if one person is constantly watering the other's garden and nurturing the relationship alone, they neglect their own garden and can become unhappy. If neither party waters the relationship's garden, it will wither and die.

- **In your relationship, do you both take responsibility for watering your own gardens as well as the relationship's garden?**

- **Does each of you put in equal amounts to the relationship's garden?**

- **Have either of you been neglecting your own garden for the sake of the relationship's garden?**

Early Relationship Lessons

Without being aware of it, we learn a great deal about relationships and communication from watching our families as we grow up. What did you learn from your family members about the following communication skills?

Communication skill	Mother/significant female	Father/significant male	Siblings/cousins/friends
Asking for what you want.			
Showing and managing feelings.			
Standing up for yourself.			
Dealing with conflict.			
Listening to and respecting others.			
Keeping the peace and conflict resolution.			

Communication Roadblocks

Do you ever find yourself falling into the following traps when trying to communicate with another and it just isn't working?

MENTAL ARGUING
No matter how well you might be appearing to listen to another, if you are mentally arguing and planning your next response, you will be limiting how you hear the other person's message. This will mean that you are closed to their main points and will not be able to see things from their perspective. When they pick up on this, they will feel invalidated and will be less likely to compromise.

BE OPEN AND RESPONSIVE

CLOUDED BY EMOTION
When we are highly emotional, we cannot think clearly or react calmly and reasonably. This makes it very difficult to communicate in a calm and assertive manner. If you feel that you cannot communicate productively because of high emotion, it is your right to take some time away from the discussion to cool down and think about what is really troubling you. This will lead to a far quicker and simpler resolution.

BE REPONSIBLE FOR YOUR FEELINGS

LACK OF CLARITY
Before you raise an issue with another, take some time to think it through. Be very clear about what the issue is for you and what you see as the best outcome. Be prepared to compromise. This will mean that you present it to the other in a clear and rational manner, therefore making a positive outcome far more likely.

BE CLEAR AND CONCISE

DEFENSIVENESS
When we feel attacked we become defensive. However, sometimes the other person is not attacking, but we interpret their actions in this way. Be aware of your own defences.

KNOW YOUR OWN ISSUES

AGGRESSION
When communicating with others, especially during conflict, it can be easy to become aggressive. Name calling, sarcasm, and belittling are forms of aggression, just like yelling and violence. All forms of aggression will sever communication, either by intimidating or by inflaming the other. Stay calm, take time out if you need to, and resume discussion when all parties are calm.

BE CALM AND RESPECTFUL

6.2 Assertiveness

In this section, clients are introduced to the concept of assertiveness. This is done through questionnaires, tip sheets and self-reflection activities all with the aim of helping the therapist to explain and practise the assertiveness skills with their clients. These activities aim to make assertiveness easily attainable for all and as non-threatening as possible.

Passive, Assertive, Aggressive

This is an information sheet that explains the difference between passive, assertive and aggressive communication styles. It explores each of these three communication modes and looks at the advantages and disadvantages of each. This sheet provides a non-threatening platform for discussion about a client's particular interaction style and areas they need to work on.

Fight–Flight

This activity uses a simple questionnaire to determine the client's predominant approach to communication (whether they are prone to fight or to flight). The items in the questionnaire provide interesting information for the therapist to discuss with the client about communication, as well as highlighting their individual communication style. This exercise increases the client's insight into their own interpersonal style and the interpretations they place on conflict.

Assertiveness

This information sheet explains the concept of assertiveness and its benefits. It also presents some suggestions for increasing assertive behaviour that could be discussed and practised in therapy. Assertive skills such as 'I' statements and how to maintain assertive body language are highlighted.

Groundrules for Assertive Behaviour

This sheet lists some important groundrules for maintaining assertive behaviour. This is a convenient checklist for the client when preparing an assertive message but is also useful as a reflective tool, because it asks the client how they feel about carrying out each assertive groundrule. This allows the therapist to pinpoint areas of difficulty with assertion and for discussion to take place.

Assertive Words

This sheet contains assertive words and phrases to demonstrate for the client how to construct assertive messages. It aims simply to prompt the client to use assertive language when expressing their opinions and beliefs. This could be used in session as part of a role-play where the therapist asks the client to construct an assertive message about a relevant topic (the client's feelings about a particular issue). Alternatively, the client could select some phrases from this sheet and add some of their own to make their own assertiveness reminder sheet.

Speaking my Mind

In this exercise, the client is asked about their feelings relating to assertiveness. This provides an opportunity for the client and therapist to talk about the fears and obstacles that might prevent the client from being assertive. This may uncover underlying beliefs stemming from family of origin and past experiences that may serve to block a client from being assertive.

Saying 'NO'

This sheet explores the concept of saying 'no' and setting limits with others. It asks the client to think about their reactions to saying 'no' and their beliefs about the consequences of this. It investigates the client's feelings about making excuses and the need for a valid reason to be saying 'no' to another. This can lead to meaningful discussion about pressures and expectations and the desire to please others. The sheet concludes with some simple suggestions for saying 'no' that could be practised or used as springboards for the generation of other examples.

Passive, Assertive, Aggressive

Passive communication involves not expressing your needs or wants and putting others first. It is characterised by avoidance of conflict and meek and non-threatening behaviour, such as lack of eye-contact, quiet voice, and stooped posture. Passive people are reluctant to express opinions and show an eagerness to please others and to 'keep the peace'. Passive people rarely get their needs met and often try to convince themselves that this does not matter. However, this can lead to resentment, bottling of their frustration and to occasional explosions.

Assertive communication involves expressing your own needs and wants and standing up for your rights, but not in a manner that violates or crushes the needs and rights of others. Assertive people express themselves clearly and value their own opinions, but also listen to others and are willing to compromise to reach a conclusion that satisfies all. Assertive people have upright postures and non-threatening gestures; they are open to others and are not afraid of conflict. They deal with conflict in a calm and rational manner by hearing each person's opinion and finding win–win solutions.

Aggressive communication involves standing up for what you want, even if that means the rights of others are ignored or violated. It often includes threatening gestures, forceful and loud tone of voice and language, and sometimes involves physical aggression. Aggressive people often get what they want but often to the detriment of their interpersonal relationships. They have learned to escalate quickly and to use aggression to push their views, but can find that others get sick of this and begin to resent or fear them.

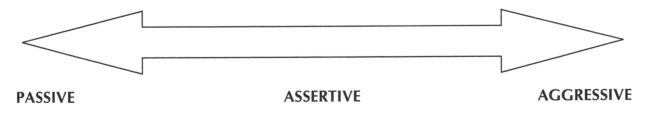

PASSIVE   **ASSERTIVE**   **AGGRESSIVE**

Passive, Assertive, Aggressive *cont.*

Assertive behaviour is a *balance* between being passive (putting your own needs last and everyone else's first) and aggressive (putting your own needs first – regardless of the consequences for others). It has more positive consequences because it involves respecting yourself and others. This improves your own self-esteem and your relationships with others.

People can use all three of these communication styles in different situations.

When are you passive?

When are you assertive?

When are you aggressive?

Fight–Flight

This questionnaire is designed to help you to understand your approach to communication with others, particularly in conflict situations.

Answer these questions as honestly as possible. You will act differently with different people and in different situations however, try to think about what you do *most of the time* when you have a problem with someone.

When you have a problem with someone, do you: (*circle*)	Rarely	Sometimes	Often	Always
explode violently	0	1	2	3
call them names	0	1	2	3
shout	0	1	2	3
interrupt them	0	1	2	3
insist you are right	0	1	2	3
talk over the other person	0	1	2	3
prove your point	0	1	2	3
argue	0	1	2	3
criticise them	0	1	2	3
threaten the other to 'do it or else'	0	1	2	3
get even	0	1	2	3
Add up your score – FIGHT TOTAL				

Fight–Flight *cont.*

Now try these questions:

When you have a problem with someone, do you: (*circle*)	Rarely	Sometimes	Often	Always
take it out on someone else	0	1	2	3
talk about them behind their back	0	1	2	3
pretend nothing is wrong	0	1	2	3
give them the 'silent treatment'	0	1	2	3
tell yourself you shouldn't be upset	0	1	2	3
dwell on how mean/bad/awful they are	0	1	2	3
withdraw from them or avoid them	0	1	2	3
get sad and upset	0	1	2	3
pretend it doesn't matter	0	1	2	3
hope the problem goes away	0	1	2	3
try to be extra nice to that person	0	1	2	3
Add up your score – FLIGHT TOTAL				

Which were you highest on – **fight** or **flight**? _____

- If you were highest on **fight**, you have a **confrontational** approach to conflict. This means that you probably get very angry and can be attacking towards others when in conflict. You like to be right and you want to win at all costs.

- If you were higher on **flight**, you have an **avoidant** approach to conflict. This means that you find conflict very uncomfortable and will do anything to prevent it. You will avoid bringing up an issue or let the other win just to keep the peace.

Assertiveness

Assertiveness is a state of mind, an attitude. It means respecting your own wants and needs enough to express them and stand up for them. Being assertive also means treating others with respect as well as yourself. You neither fight (become confrontational) nor run away (avoid) – you FLOW!

For those who FIGHT: You need to adjust how you see conflict. It is not something that you have to win at all costs, it is a chance to deepen and improve your relationships. You must tone down your approach and only speak from your perspective and feelings. Remember always to respect the other and to keep in mind that you want to keep this relationship in the future.

For those who take FLIGHT in conflict situations: It is hard for some people to speak up for themselves but it is an important part of improving your self-esteem. If you value yourself, you need to value your feelings. So if someone has done something that makes you feel uncomfortable, you owe it to yourself to speak up rather than ignoring it. Start speaking up about little things and gradually build up to more difficult things.

Assertiveness tips – how to flow

- Go away and think about what is upsetting you before you approach the other person.

- Write down what you want to say first and practise it on someone else to get their feedback.

- Use an 'I' statement to make sure you express yourself clearly and from your own perspective:

  I feel _____ (your emotion)

  when you _____ (what they do that upsets you)

  I would like _____ (what you want them to do differently)

Assertiveness *cont.*

- Ask the other person if you can talk to them – pick a time that is good for both of you – don't ambush them!

- Talk to them *alone* – don't include others.

- Remember that above all else, you want to keep this relationship and that most people wouldn't hurt your feelings on purpose.

- Remain focused that if something upsets you, you have a right to speak up about it – don't allow yourself to avoid!

- Keep your voice calm and level.

- Stick to your point, don't get sidetracked.

- Maintain good eye-contact.

- Stand up straight.

- Don't apologise for your feelings – you are allowed to have them.

- Give them the benefit of the doubt – they may not have done anything intentionally so your comments may come as a surprise.

- If they don't seem to be hearing you, repeat your message calmly and clearly and then let it go (for now!). Sometimes, people need to go away and think about it before they can fully understand your point.

Groundrules for Assertive Behaviour

GROUNDRULE	HOW I FEEL ABOUT DOING THIS
Stand up straight and maintain good eye-contact.	
Project your voice in a confident but not aggressive manner.	
Believe that your opinion is valid and worth being expressed and heard.	
Express yourself in a respectful way (no name-calling, sarcasm or threatening behaviour).	
Be prepared to repeat your message if it is not heard.	
Listen to what the other person has to say – be open to their viewpoint.	
Don't get sidetracked from the issue you wanted to raise.	
Avoid negative body language like eye-rolling, turning away or sighing.	
Be prepared to compromise.	
If the conversation seems to be escalating into aggression, ask for time out to cool down.	
Be prepared to revisit the issue until you feel satisfied that you have been acknowledged.	

Assertive Words

I believe...

I feel...

What is most important to me is...

I respect your opinion.

I hear what you are saying.

I would prefer...

What I would like...

In my opinion...

How about a compromise?

My feelings...

So what you're saying is...

Speaking my Mind

When I think about standing up for myself and being assertive I feel:

The last time I tried this:

My fears about speaking my mind are:

What things do I need to remember when I try to be assertive?

Saying 'NO'

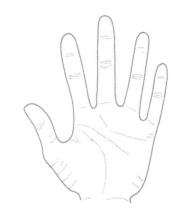

Saying 'NO' to people can be very hard, especially when you think there will be negative consequences if you say no.

If you have to say 'NO' to someone you care about, how do you feel? Why?

Do you believe that you can only say 'NO' if you have a valid reason?

Would you prefer to make up a reason, even if it's not true, than say 'NO'?

Do you think the other person has a right to be angry with you if you say 'NO' to a request they have made of you?

Do you believe that just 'not feeling like it' is a good enough reason to say 'NO'? Why?

What do you think will happen if you say 'NO' to someone?

Here are some examples of how you can say 'NO' if you need to:

- 'Thanks for thinking of me, but I won't be able to.'
- 'I'm not available, but how about next time?'
- 'No, I'd rather not.'
- 'No, that doesn't work for me.'
- 'No thanks, I'm not really into…'
- 'No, that doesn't suit me.'
- 'No, I have other plans.'

6.3 Conflict resolution

This is an area of communication that many adults find daunting and may need assistance with. The following exercises combine self-exploration with skills training to help improve clients' assertiveness and confidence in their approach to conflict.

Conflict Styles

This table outlines five different styles of dealing with conflict, including the avoider, the peacemaker, the confronter, the compromiser and the collaborator. This will help clients to understand different people's approaches to conflict, as well as their own. It might help them to discuss with the therapist their own favoured style and the styles of those in their life.

Conflict Resolution

This information sheet provides the steps of conflict resolution as well as important assertiveness tips to remember during conflict situations. This might aid role-playing in session, or preparation to deal with a difficult issue in the client's life.

Keeping Communication open during Conflict

This sheet asks clients to think about the things that they or the other person in a conflict could do to keep communication open or to close communication down. The aim of this exercise is to highlight the importance of remaining calm and assertive during conflict resolution in order to reach a satisfactory solution. It does this by emphasising how destructive certain communication strategies (yelling, interrupting, name-calling) can be to the outcome of conflict.

Mapping the Conflict

This sheet shows how to look at a conflict from many sides to determine the needs, fears and wants of all involved parties. It shows clients how to take a broad perspective on conflict and to consider the stance of all others involved. This can be very effective for creating empathy and understanding towards others and for empowering clients to find solutions to complex interpersonal problems.

Conflict

This sheet explores what conflict means to the client. It touches on the client's early experiences with conflict, their beliefs about conflict, and their current approach to conflict. This is a valuable therapeutic tool for work with clients suffering from a range of interpersonal issues.

Mediation

This tip sheet explains the process of mediation and the role of the mediator. It might be a useful tool for teaching a client how to mediate among work colleagues, friends or family members. Mediation combines the skills of assertiveness and conflict resolution, so might be a good revision task for assertiveness training.

Conflict Styles

Below are listed some different ways that people resolve conflict situations involving other people. Which do you think applies to you?

CONFLICT STYLE	REASONING	ADVANTAGES	DISADVANTAGES
THE AVOIDER	'If I ignore it, the problem will go away.' 'There is no problem here!'	Avoids negative interactions with others. Others get their own way, so usually like the avoider. Prevents possible conflict over small things.	The avoider can be walked over by others and never addresses the issues that might be important to them. Some problems will not go away.
THE PEACEMAKER	'Let's keep everyone happy.' 'I'm sure we can all fix this together.'	The peacemaker wants everyone to be happy and emphasises harmony. Smooths over small issues.	This approach can 'gloss' over bigger issues in its attempt to hastily make the peace. It can create the illusion of problem-solving.
THE CONFRONTER	'Let's talk about what's really going on here.' 'I can't believe you...'	The confronter likes to get all problems out in the open, no matter how painful. This can get to the bottom of an issue and clear the air.	Can be controlling and intimidating, causing hidden resentment in others and sometimes leading to blocking of resolution.
THE COMPROMISER	'How can we make everyone happy?' 'Can we find some common ground?'	Tries to meet all parties' needs in some way by giving each person some of what they wanted.	Can mean that no-one ends up happy and the problem is still unresolved. Puts all the responsibility for solving the problem onto the compromiser and not the group.
THE COLLABORATOR	'Let's hear from each person.' 'What do we see as possible solutions?'	Lets each person express their concerns and possible solutions. All feel heard and all contribute to solving the problem. The problem is aired and solved collaboratively.	Can challenge existing power structures because the group becomes powerful in its own right with no clear leader needed.

Conflict Resolution

When dealing with a conflict situation, it is important that you choose to **RESPOND** rather than **REACT**. Responding means that you think things through and you respond to the conflict in a constructive and assertive manner. Reacting means that you approach the conflict in an automatic, defensive manner implying that it is something threatening and frightening.

Try to respond to conflict by:

- managing your emotions: **BREATHE AND RELAX**

- saying nothing at first: **LISTEN AND BE OPEN**

- focusing on the facts: **CONCENTRATE**

- ignoring inflammatory remarks: **DON'T BE DEFENSIVE**

- when they have stated their case: **PARAPHRASE to CLARIFY**

- stating your opinion: **BE CALM AND ASSERTIVE**

- describing your wants, needs and feelings: **YOU HAVE A RIGHT TO BE HEARD**

- being prepared to **COMPROMISE** and to work together to find a **SOLUTION**

- remember that both parties are responsible for resolving this issue.

How do you feel about carrying out these steps to resolve conflict?

What seems easy? Why?

What seems difficult? Why?

Keeping Communication open during Conflict

List some of the things that you or the other person could do to in a conflict situation to:

OPEN UP COMMUNICATION	CLOSE DOWN COMMUNICATION

Mapping the Conflict

Who: _____
Needs: _____
_____
_____
Fears: _____
_____
_____
Wants: _____

Who: _____
Needs: _____
_____
_____
Fears: _____
_____
_____
Wants: _____

THE PROBLEM
_____
_____
_____
_____
_____
_____
_____

Who: _____
Needs: _____
_____
_____
Fears: _____
_____
_____
Wants: _____

Who: _____
Needs: _____
_____
_____
Fears: _____
_____
_____
Wants: _____

Conflict

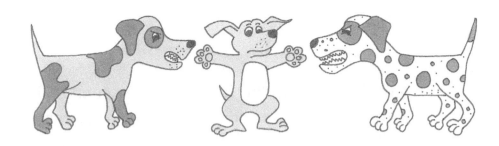

When you think about conflict, what words, feelings, and images come to mind?

As a child, what were your experiences with conflict?

How do you deal with conflict as an adult?

What do you believe about conflict?

Mediation

To be an effective mediator between people in conflict, it is important to remain neutral and to be focused on finding an adequate outcome for all parties involved. Tho do this, the mediator needs to follow these steps:

1. Set rules

a. Before *anyone* starts to speak, the mediator needs to define their role and set some groundrules for how this discussion will go.

b. They need to firstly explain that they are on no-one's side and that no-one is right or wrong, that all people are entitled to their feelings but that they must be expressed appropriately.

c. Set clear rules about no interrupting, name-calling, or blaming. People are to speak ONE AT A TIME and to LISTEN to each other.

d. Then, the mediator needs to make it clear to all parties that a solution must be found to the problem so that they can all move on.

e. The mediator may need to remind everyone that they will have to be willing to compromise to reach a solution.

2. Listen to everyone

a. Now it is time for the mediator to invite each person to explain their feelings in relation to the issue. This is to be done in a constructive and assertive manner. The mediator may have to pause them if they become aggressive or overly emotive.

b. The mediator may need to reinforce that everyone's opinion is valid and deserves to be heard.

c. Once each person has had time to express their needs, the mediator paraphrases each person's perspective non-judgementally to clarify that they heard them correctly. This allows the other parties to hear each person's viewpoint twice.

d. Make sure that all listen and do not interrupt, argue or judge.

e. If necessary, it can be useful to have each person paraphrase the other's viewpoint as well, so that all demonstrate an understanding of each other.

3. Resolve the conflict

a. In the third stage, the mediator guides each person to make a suggestion to resolve the conflict. All must be responsible for trying to solve the problem and therefore, must contribute.

b. It is important that the mediator reminds all people that compromise and understanding are important in resolving conflict, and not to judge suggestions before considering all options.

c. The mediator then guides a discussion about the advantages and disadvantages of each suggestion and helps an agreement to be reached.

d. All involved parties must commit to the agreement and then plan how to execute it.

6.4 Social skills

Being able to converse comfortably with others is a skill with which some clients may need assistance. The following section covers several basic social skills and can be used to coach clients through the process of social skills training. The worksheets included cover one skill each and could be used to teach the client before role-playing and practising the particular conversation skills in vivo.

Checklist for Positive Interaction

This checklist illustrates the verbal and nonverbal cues necessary for positive communication with others. It outlines how to appear open to interaction and how to maintain a positive, confident and welcoming stance when first meeting others. This is useful for clients who become very anxious about social interaction and believe that all around them can detect their fear.

Small Talk

This exercise asks the client to think about their fears regarding small talk, that is, making light conversation with new people in a controlled setting such as a work or social function. Some conversation starters are provided and space allowed for the client and/or the therapist to generate some other suggestions for conversation starters that might be relevant to the types of settings the client is likely to encounter. It is beneficial for the client to role-play these conversation starters with the therapist to increase their confidence.

Feared Situations

This sheet allows the client to list any social situations that they feel uncomfortable in and avoid. This provides the therapist with useful information regarding the client's social activities and their level of avoidance. If necessary, these situations might become therapeutic goals and form part of an exposure therapy hierarchy to help the client to overcome their anxiety in these situations.

Advanced Social Skills 1

This sheet describes the advanced social skill of joining established conversations. This skill is a vital small talk skill and often causes people some level of anxiety. Discussing and practising joining conversations might reduce the client's fears about these situations, so improving their social confidence.

Advanced Social Skills 2

This sheet describes two more advanced social skills, including changing topics of conversation and coping with silences. These skills build upon the skill described in Advanced Social Skills 1. By discussing and role-playing these skills, clients can significantly reduce their anxiety about social and small talk situations.

Advanced Social Skills 3

This sheet describes two final advanced social skills, including accepting compliments and conveying sympathy. The client's fears about encountering these situations can be reduced by discussing and practising these skills.

Checklist for Positive Interaction

When you first meet other people, try the following ideas to help yourself to appear confident, relaxed and approachable.

- **Stand up straight.** Your posture instantly gives others an impression about your confidence.

- **Smile!** If you look welcoming and friendly, others will seek you out and respond positively to you.

- **Manage your feelings**. If situations where you have to first meet people and make small talk make you nervous, breathe calmly and slowly and tell yourself that you are going to be fine.

- **Have a few 'conversation starters'** ready to open up conversation.

- **Make eye-contact** with the speaker and encourage them by nodding and asking questions.

- **Listen!** Concentrate on their main points. This may lead to further topics of conversation or questions.

- **Don't focus on your thoughts** ('Oh no! What am I going to say next?'). Instead, listen to the other and let conversation happen.

Which of these skills do you already use?

Which of these skills do you need to practise?

Small Talk

Making light conversation with people you hardly know can be an uncomfortable task. However, being able to do this is an important part of social interaction. Luckily, this is a skill that can be learned.

What is the worst thing about making small talk?

How do you normally make small talk?

Small Talk *cont.*

The key is to look more confident than you feel and to have some questions ready to ask. This takes the focus off you and allows you to listen.

Try some of these conversation starters:

- 'Hi, I'm Margaret! How are you?'

- 'What do you do for work?'

- 'How do you know Bob?'

- 'How's your work/family?'

- 'How do you spend your weekends?'

- 'Have you been on holidays recently?'

- 'Have you seen any good movies lately?'

Now you try to think of some conversation starters that would be appropriate to a small-talk setting you are likely to encounter:

Feared Situations

List below any social situation you feel uncomfortable in and what it is about that situation that makes you anxious:

Social situation	What makes it uncomfortable?

Advanced Social Skills 1

Joining conversations

- In a social setting, it can seem very difficult to join into already established conversations. However, if you don't attempt to join in, you may find it difficult to talk to anyone!

- First, assess the conversations going on around you. Pick one to join where you know some of the people, or failing that, a conversation that does not look too personal or overly familiar. It is much harder (and sometimes not welcome) to join a group of people who know each other very well.

- Pick a group that seems relatively unfamiliar and that forms a loose circle, rather than a tight circle where everyone is leaning in to talk. This will make it easier for you to join in without having to push your way in!

- Approach the group and briefly 'hover' on the outskirts and wait to see if you receive eye-contact from any of the members. As soon as you do, you're in! Step a little into the circle to join, and the people alongside you should open the circle to allow you in by turning their shoulders slightly towards you.

- If you do not receive eye-contact and the circle does not open, it is best to quit while you are ahead and move on to another group, rather than pushing to join this one.

- Once in a group, smile and politely listen to the conversation until you think you could contribute something. Don't try to take over, just add something. Be sure to smile and introduce yourself when the opportunity arises.

Advanced Social Skills 2

Changing topics of conversation

- If you have managed to make adequate small talk with someone at a social function for some time and the topic of conversation enters an area that makes you feel uncomfortable, being able to seamlessly change topics is a valuable skill. It is vital that you do not talk about things that make you feel uncomfortable just for the sake of conversation. This will leave you feeling exposed and unhappy afterwards.

- To change topics well, it is important that the other person does not feel rebuked or that you do not want to talk to them anymore. Try a more subtle topic change first, like: 'I am interested in hearing more about…' or 'I'd rather talk about…' If they persist, then you might need to be more clear by saying 'I'm not really comfortable talking about that,' or 'Let's not talk about such a depressing topic!'

- This works best if you are pleasant but firm and redirect conversation into other areas by asking the other person a question about themselves.

Coping with silences

- When making conversation at a social gathering, many people fear silences and their accompanying awkwardness. For coping with silences, it is important to remember that silence is a normal part of conversation and that it is not all your responsibility to produce the conversation.

- If you have some questions ready to ask the other and you look interested in the conversation, then you have fulfilled your responsibility. This means that any silences are a dual responsibility and not 100 per cent up to you to 'fix'.

- If silences occur, use them as a time to think, to look around and to wait for the other to speak! If you try to fill in any silence, you may actually be cutting off the other person before they begin to speak, and therefore missing an opportunity to listen rather than talk (and we know that this is much easier than speaking!).

Advanced Social Skills 3

Accepting compliments

- Accepting compliments graciously is a valuable and necessary social skill that, unfortunately, most people struggle with. When someone offers you a compliment they are offering you a gift. To refuse it or brush it off is extremely invalidating. Think about when you give someone a compliment: do you mean it? How would it feel to have that compliment (no matter how small) rejected?

- Accepting a compliment does not make you 'full of yourself' or arrogant. It makes you gracious towards the other and towards yourself. Letting compliments in and believing them are vital tasks for the development of healthy self-esteem.

- Next time you receive a compliment, try saying 'Thank-you' and believing it.

Conveying sympathy

- Conveying appropriate sympathy when someone around you is grieving can be a delicate matter and one that many people avoid, for fear of upsetting the person.

- When conveying sympathy, remember that you do not have to say the 'perfect' thing because there are no perfect sentiments to be expressed.

- Generally, any expression of acknowledgment is preferable to avoiding the issue or pretending nothing is wrong. Be careful not to try to solve the problem for the other or to 'cheer them up'. Simply show them that you care and that you are there for them.

- For example, you could say 'I can't imagine what this is like for you, but I can listen if you need to talk,' or 'Let me know if there is anything I can do to help.'

DESSERT

7 SELF-ESTEEM

7.1 Psycho-education

Having a healthy self-esteem is vital for an individual's development and wellbeing. High self-esteem makes people more resilient, more positive and more contented in life. This section contains information sheets about self-esteem and self-awareness and some exercises to clarify these concepts. The information in this first section is predominantly psycho-educational.

Self-esteem

This is an information sheet about self-esteem that explains what it is, how it develops, and why self-esteem is important to have. It is useful for early psycho-education about this concept.

Factors that Affect Self-esteem

In this information sheet, the factors that impact upon a person's level of self-esteem are outlined. Suggestions are given regarding increasing self-esteem, and what things can decrease a person's self-esteem. This may be useful for the client to take away to think about the concept of self-esteem.

What is Self-esteem?

This is an alternative exercise to the two previous information sheets, and could be given initially to elicit thought about self-esteem before reading the information sheets. This might assist the therapist to ascertain the client's level of understanding about self-esteem as a concept before entering into psycho-education.

Self-awareness

This sheet explains how to be self-aware and guides the client through some exercises to explore a little about themselves. This activity might assist the therapist by emphasising the importance of self-awareness and encouraging the client to begin the process of self-exploration.

Increasing Self-esteem

This is a list of strategies to increase self-esteem. It might be useful for providing ideas for the client, as well as being a springboard for other ideas generated by the client and the therapist. Many people feel powerless to increase their self-esteem, so this sheet intends to remove some of the mystery surrounding this concept by providing practical suggestions for activities that help to increase self-esteem.

Self-esteem

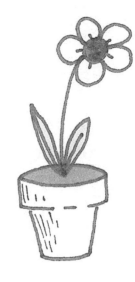

What is self-esteem?

Self-esteem is your self-image (how you see yourself) or how you feel about yourself. It is an ongoing opinion you develop throughout your life that is made up of thoughts and feelings. You may have a positive, neutral or negative opinion of yourself. Sometimes people are not really aware of how they feel about themselves.

Self-esteem affects the way you think, act and feel about yourself and others.

Where does it come from?

Your self-esteem grows like a plant. If it is nurtured and cared for, it will flourish and be able to weather blows. However, if it is depleted and mistreated, it will be stunted in its growth and very fragile.

Self-esteem comes from two sources: *yourself* and your *environment*. Let's start with your **environment**. All your experiences with other people in your life shape the way you view yourself. Your family environment, school, work, and social lives all teach you lessons about yourself and where you fit as a person. The culture and society you are raised in teaches you about how you should look and act in order to be accepted. All of these parts of your life affect your self-esteem.

Second, your self-esteem comes from **within you**. It involves knowing yourself and accepting yourself as an OK person – *flaws and all*. It comes from your perception of your own control over who you are and the choices you make.

Why is it good to have?

Self-esteem is important because if you feel good about yourself, you will be confident, relaxed and assertive with yourself and others. You will feel less pressure to be something you are not. You will follow your dreams because you will believe in yourself. You will be less sensitive to criticism and better able to bounce back from disappointment. You will accept the fact that no-one is perfect and you will not expect yourself to be.

Therefore, you will be kinder to yourself and others. You will be confident enough to stand up for what you believe in and be less influenced by others. You won't make yourself unhappy as a result of self-criticism.

Factors that Affect Self-esteem

How could you improve your self-esteem?

- Accept that you are who you are (even if you're not sure who that is yet!). You are unique and special just as you are.

- Remind yourself that no-one is perfect and that you don't need to be. Focus on your strengths, remind yourself of them every day!

- Allow yourself to be drawn to people who make you feel good about yourself. Steer clear of people who criticise you or make you feel as if you should be someone else.

- Reward yourself when you do something well.

- Be kind to yourself – be your own best friend.

- Accept compliments!

- Take on challenges and be proud of what you achieve.

- Forgive yourself for your mistakes – we all make mistakes, and without them we would not learn. Don't dwell on your imperfections or disappointments.

What things decrease a person's self-esteem?

- Self-criticism is probably the most damaging thing to a person's self-esteem. Whether this self-criticism was started by others or was your own initiative, it deflates your self-esteem, taking with it your positive feelings, confidence and motivation.

- Negative, critical people who make you feel that you are not good enough as you are can be a huge drain on your self-esteem as well. Encouragement is positive but criticism is detrimental to self-esteem.

- Expecting yourself to be perfect also lowers self-esteem because it is unrealistic and sets you up to feel bad about yourself.

- Putting yourself last through ignoring your own feelings, dreams, goals, and opinions decreases your self-esteem and can lead to resentment.

- Denying yourself of opportunities to shine reduces self-esteem.

What is Self-esteem?

What is self-esteem?

Where does it come from?

Why is it good to have?

How could you increase your self-esteem?

What things decrease a persons' self-esteem?

Self-awareness

Being self-aware means knowing yourself, including your:

- opinions

- feelings

- dreams and desires

- fears

- habits

- strengths

- faults

- interests

- behaviour

- likes and dislikes

- history

- stressors.

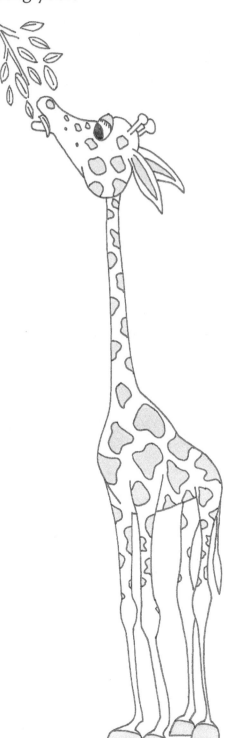

Being self-aware increases your sense of centeredness, identity and self-acceptance.

It makes it easier to make good decisions for yourself and to be responsible for those decisions.

It helps you to understand and manage your feelings and actions.

Self-awareness helps you to set realistic goals because you know your own limitations and expectations.

How well do you know yourself?

In which areas do you feel that you need to get to know yourself better?

VISUALISATION

Take a few moments to visualise a place that makes you feel perfectly comfortable and at peace... What does it look like...feel like...smell like? What are the surroundings? What sounds are there? Which people would you have in your special place?

Why is this place special to you?

What does it tell you about yourself?

Increasing Self-esteem

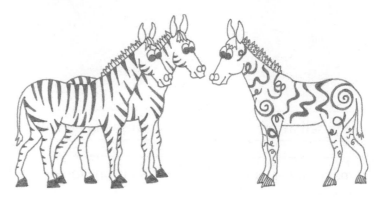

Try to do something to increase your self-esteem every day! Try some of these ideas to improve your self-liking, confidence and general sense of wellbeing.

- Acknowledge your strengths, achievements and successes.
- Work on improving yourself by setting personal goals, but learn to accept some of your flaws.
- Cherish your uniqueness.
- Do not expect perfection from yourself or others.
- Make time to completely please yourself.
- Express your own feelings and opinions.
- Remember and cherish the compliments given to you.
- Appreciate the things you do *well* – not perfectly.
- Set goals and make achieving them a priority for yourself.
- Be kind to yourself.
- Prioritise your own needs some of the time.
- Treat yourself to something special.
- Have realistic expectations for yourself and celebrate your progress.
- Expect others to treat you with respect.
- Think positively about yourself.
- Let negativity and criticism wash over you but not overwhelm you.
- Learn from your mistakes and try again.
- Stop criticising or blaming yourself – this only erodes your self-esteem.
- Do one thing a day that you enjoy.
- Seek out others who affirm you and who make you feel good about yourself.
- Stand up for yourself if others violate your rights.
- Have fun, enjoy life, enjoy being you – just as you are.

7.2 Self-awareness

This section aims to encourage clients to explore themselves in order to increase their sense of self-awareness, centeredness and identity. The activities are very much exploratory and are designed to encourage clients to reflect upon themselves, their beliefs, dreams and opinions.

The Ins and Outs of Me

This exercise encourages clients to think deeply about themselves and to explore their deepest desires, fears and dreams. This is useful for helping people to become more familiar with themselves and for gaining an increased sense of self-awareness. The therapist could guide this process to the appropriate level of self-exploration and discovery and perhaps use this as a tool to elicit deeper conversation.

My Personality

This sheet asks the client to reflect upon their personality traits and to rate themselves on several polarised scales. This promotes self-awareness and might lead to discussion about each personality trait. This exercise could uncover the client's deeper opinions and beliefs about their personality and provide opportunity for personal reflection and challenging by the therapist.

My Opinions

This activity asks clients to share some of their opinions regarding things that are important to them. This aims to help them to explore their feelings and opinions in an atmosphere of acceptance and understanding. This is intended to be affirming of the client's individuality and legitimacy, while helping them to increase their self-awareness.

My Assets

This sheet encourages clients to look at themselves through another's eyes and to see the assets that others notice in them. This can help clients to remove some of their own self-criticism and judgement and to really see themselves objectively. This leads on to ways for enhancing self-esteem in the next section.

The Ins and Outs of Me

This is a worksheet to help you explore a bit about who you are and what your beliefs are. The first step to improving your self-esteem is to get to know yourself.

What did you enjoy doing as a child that you do not do now?

What would you do if you knew you couldn't fail?

What interest or passion have you never pursued or told anyone about?

What do you dream about that you never express? What is your wildest dream?

What would you regret not having done if your life was ending?

My Personality

Rate yourself by marking on the line where you fit:

Funny	_____	Serious
Dishonest	_____	Honest
Keeps promises	_____	Breaks promises
Sad	_____	Happy
Impatient	_____	Patient
Active	_____	Passive
Bossy	_____	Easy-going
Tense	_____	Relaxed
People-person	_____	Loner
Quiet	_____	Loud
Positive	_____	Negative
Worrier	_____	Laid-back
Confident	_____	Unsure
Messy	_____	Tidy
Organised	_____	Disorganised
Reliable	_____	Unreliable
Leader	_____	Team member
Aggressive	_____	Submissive
Sporty	_____	Not sporty
Express feelings	_____	Bottle feelings
Stand up for self	_____	Don't stand up for self
Compare self to others	_____	Don't compare

My Opinions

Three things I feel strongly about are:

1.

2.

3.

Injustice to me means _____

_____

_____

If I could **change the world** _____

_____

_____

What do you think the world will be like in 100 years' time? _____

_____

_____

My Assets

How do others see you? How would they describe you to someone who doesn't know you?

What things do others compliment you on?

What I acknowledge as some of my assets:

A challenge I have overcome in my life:

7.3 Increasing self-esteem

This section contains worksheets and activities for clients to help them to increase their self-esteem. As an experience that most could benefit from, enhancing self-esteem is a process that takes time. These sheets aim to expedite the process for clients, as well as providing therapists with many ideas and a variety of resources for helping their clients to develop in this area.

Good Things about ME!

This exercise is similar to the previous one but focuses a little more on achievements and specific positive personality traits of the client. If encouragement is needed, the following sheet, 'Positive Traits', may provide prompts for personality qualities. Clients are encouraged to read through this sheet daily to help them to acknowledge their positive qualities.

Positive Traits

This is an exhaustive list of positive personality traits that could provide suggestions of positive qualities that clients possess. It is important that clients learn how to acknowledge their positive qualities even if they do not possess those qualities 'all of the time'. It is vital that they learn that they do not have to wait until they are 'perfect' to praise themselves. Therapist could enlarge this sheet and cut out each positive trait so that the client could sort through the pile, identifying those positive traits that they feel that they possess, as well as those that they would like to increase.

My Achievements!

This is an unstructured sheet to allow the client to record their life's achievements. This allows discussion and validation of success, no matter how large or small. Many clients have difficulty with this task and may need some encouragement from the therapist. Such difficulty allows for discussion about why the client finds it so hard to praise themselves and to celebrate their successes (particularly when people find it so easy to be critical of themselves).

Be Kind to Yourself!

This is a tip sheet for increasing self-esteem. It contains practical suggestions and cautions for clients. Clients often need constant reminders to treat themselves the way they treat others.

My Successes

This activity is designed to encourage clients to review their successes throughout their lifespan, as well as thinking about something they would like to achieve in the future.

Challenging Self-criticism

This sheet highlights the effect of negative and self-critical thinking on self-esteem by asking clients to record their self-critical thinking and its subsequent effect on their feelings and behaviour. Clients are then asked to change this critical thinking into more helpful and productive thoughts that can help to build rather than deplete self-esteem.

Good Things about ME!

Focusing on your strengths is the best way to increase your self-esteem. List below four things you have done that you are proud of:

-
-
-
-

Write in below some of your positive traits. Don't be shy – remember this is healthy for your self-esteem!

Stick this sheet on your bathroom/bedroom mirror and read it every day!

Positive Traits

pleasant	strong	brave	honest
unique	trustworthy	polite	wanted
tidy	interested	caring	trusting
talented	easy-going	imaginative	dependable
forgiving	interesting	tolerant	patient
charming	funny	out-going	social
warm	giving	gentle	determined
dedicated	affectionate	sensitive	fair
good sport	team player	leader	helpful
enthusiastic	sincere	open	good friend
original	ambitious	flexible	intelligent
listener	serious	cautious	realistic
independent	energetic	entertaining	open-minded
adventurous	hard worker	positive	co-operative
self-confident	assertive	creative	fun
loyal	friendly	inclusive	consistent
generous	truthful	quiet	accepting
thoughtful	punctual	focused	calm
self-starter	selfless	risk-taker	daring
bold	moral	nurturing	problem-solver
playful	driven	respectful	special
kind	mature	loving	confident
logical	rational	reliable	spontaneous

My Achievements!

Be Kind to Yourself!

Follow these steps to increase your self-esteem:

PRAISE YOURSELF!

- Acknowledge your good qualities.
- Value your successes.
- Focus on your strengths.

SPEAK NICELY TO YOURSELF!

- Stop self-criticism.
- Do not call yourself names!

ACCEPT COMPLIMENTS!

- Let compliments in and bask in them.
- Do not brush them off.
- Say "Thank-you."

LEARN FROM MISTAKES!

- Don't beat yourself up, learn and try again.
- Your behaviors are separate from you.

VALUE YOUR NEEDS!

- Consider your own needs and wants sometimes!
- Own your feelings, behaviors and opinions.

STOP FEELING GUILTY AND INADEQUATE!

- You are OK just as you are, flaws and all!
- Cherish and love yourself.

My Successes

Think of a success that you had during the following stages of your life:

Before school

Primary school

High school

As an adult

In the past month

Something you would like to achieve in the future

Challenging Self-criticism

List below some of the negative things you say to yourself that erodes your self-esteem.

Self-critical thoughts	Consequences	Alternative thought
What you say to yourself	How does that thought make you feel about yourself? How does it make you behave?	Think of a more helpful and realistic thought that could replace the critical one.

SECTION 8 RESILIENCE

8.1 Staying positive

This section focuses on staying positive, no matter what life throws at you. A range of techniques for helping clients to remain positive are illustrated in this section. These activities encourage clients to acknowledge and cherish the positive in their lives.

Mantras

This sheet lists several mantras or motivational sayings that could inspire clients to remain positive and focused on their goals. It aims to prompt clients to think positively and to believe in positive outcomes in their lives. The examples on this sheet could lead the client to generate mantras of their own, to be used whenever they find themselves thinking negatively.

Some activities that could arise from this sheet are for the therapist and client to select a mantra (or create a unique one) and to create an artwork featuring it, make it into a motivational poster, or record it with background music to be played while the client relaxes.

Affirmations – Coping Statements

This sheet allows the client to record some positive affirmations and coping statements onto cue cards to carry with them. This means that the most meaningful positive thoughts that have been generated from cognitive restructuring or from therapist challenging can be placed on these cards to prompt the client to challenge their negative thinking each time it occurs. This helps the client to 'unlearn' their negative thinking by replacing it each time with positive, realistic thoughts.

Cheap Thrills

This sheet lists many of the beautiful and wonderful things that often go unnoticed in day-to-day life. This list aims to open the client's eyes to the good around them and to encourage them to see the things that make them feel positive about their lives, which they might not recognise or appreciate. This can lead to meaningful discussion with clients about what matters to them in their lives, the things they appreciate and the small things that give them a lift when they are feeling sad. This teaches clients to see the positive around them rather than focusing on the negative.

Gratitude

This exercise encourages the client to acknowledge the things they are grateful for in their life and could be launched from the previous sheet (Cheap Thrills). This leads the client to recognise the positive in their life and to use this to help them through the times when they feel down, disheartened or unsure of themselves.

Mantras

I am OK just as I am.

I have the right to feel, to want, and to be treated with respect.

I choose to be happy.

This too shall pass.

I am strong.

I have coped before, I will cope again.

My feelings are valid.

I deserve to be content.

I can manage the challenges of life.

Limitations are merely opportunities to grow.

I refuse to be helpless – I am powerful.

I will no longer wait for myself to be perfect in order to love myself.

I am in control of my own life and my own happiness

Breathe and relax.

Nothing is worth worrying about to the extent that it stops me from living life now.

Mistakes lead to learning.

I am surrounded by people who love me.

I let go of all negativity in my life.

I can find to solutions to my problems.

Thinking positively helps me to become positive.

The more I learn, the more I grow.

Affirmations – Coping Statements

**Affirmations – coping
statements**

_____

_____

_____

_____

_____

_____

_____

**Affirmations – coping
statements**

_____

_____

_____

_____

_____

_____

_____

**Affirmations – coping
statements**

_____

_____

_____

_____

_____

_____

_____

**Affirmations – coping
statements**

_____

_____

_____

_____

_____

_____

_____

Cheap Thrills

singing, dancing, sleeping, yelling, moving, watching the sun set, listening to bird song, smelling cookies baking, babies' soft skin, lying on the grass, early morning air, eating, running, breathing, hugging, beautiful music, puppies' bellies, looking forward to something, lying in a hot bath, massage, reading, walking, gardening, jumping, smelling freshly cut lawn, listening to rain on the roof, watching storms roll in, laughing, playing, movies, talking, sharing, diving into cool water, listening to a child giggle, warm jumpers on cold days, open fires, feeling at one with nature, friends, watching waves lap the shore, telling someone you love them, listening to rivers burbling, excitement in the pit of your stomach, a great idea, staring at the night sky, completing something, climbing trees, family, digging your feet into sand, fixing something, creating, cool breezes on hot days, marvelling at others' creations, smiles from strangers, long lazy days, understanding, breakfast in bed, walking on a beach, lying on the floor of a forest, making shapes out of clouds, sharing your deepest thoughts with another, feeling loved, stroking a cat's back, being captivated by the perfection of a single flower, seeing your breath on frosty mornings, holding hands, beautiful music, riding down a hill fast on a bicycle, new beginnings, doing something for someone else and expecting nothing in return, holidays, staying in your pyjamas all day, treating yourself to something you really want but don't need, cooking a nice meal, sighing, bubble baths, looking at old photos, planning a party, writing and reading poetry, listening, chocolate, quiet, being close to others, peace, challenging yourself, rewarding yourself

Gratitute

Write below some of the things you are grateful for in your life and why:

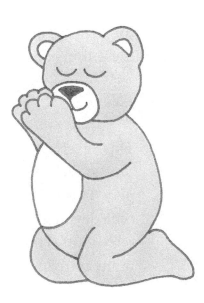

8.2 Managing stress

Coping with stress is very important for general resilience and satisfaction with life. This section aims to introduce some practical stress management and organisational skills to help to train clients to manage stress and stay in control of their lives.

Stress Management

This sheet explains some of the things that cause stress and how to reduce stress in your life. It is an educational sheet that might help to guide treatment goals and improve the client's understanding of stress and how to reduce it.

De-stressing your Thinking

This sheet lists some strategies for managing stress by changing perfectionistic thought patterns that could be contributing to a client's stress level. This would particularly suit clients with high standards for their own performance and with negative self-talk that fuels their stress levels.

Things that Cause me Stress...

This exercise encourages the client to reflect upon the things that cause them stress in their lives and to think about how much control they have over these things. This could open up discussion about personal power and the client's perception of control over the things they can and can't change. It also leads to discussion about the benefits of changing their responses to the things they cannot control so that these things do not cause them so much distress.

Balance

This sheet aims to make the client think about the different ways they spend their time and to see whether they feel that they have a balance between work, rest and play. This enables the therapist and the client to review objectively the amount of time devoted to stress-inducing areas of the client's life, as well as to relaxation and recreation. This may lead to goal-setting for pleasant activities and the setting of limits to reduce the time spent in stress-inducing activities.

Relaxation and Balance

In this activity, the client is first encouraged to reflect on how much relaxation they engage in on a regular basis. Second, they are asked to list relaxing activities that they would like to participate in. Finally, they are asked to think about which activities they could do daily, weekly and monthly to ensure that relaxing and pleasant activities form a regular part of their lifestyle. It is important that the therapist stresses the reasons for relaxation and makes the client think about the benefits of each activity as they list them. This will increase the client's motivation to carry out each relaxing activity without brushing it aside.

Stress Management

Stress is a normal reaction to the demands placed upon you. In moderate doses, stress can be positive because it can motivate you to get things done (i.e. deadlines) or to perform well (i.e. in sports). However, stress in higher levels becomes unhealthy because it reduces your performance and your ability to cope with the demands placed upon you. Prolonged levels of high stress can be harmful to your physical and mental health.

The feeling of stress and its symptoms let you know when the pressures on you are beginning to exceed your ability to cope with them. All people respond to pressure and experience stress slightly differently.

Some of the symptoms of stress:

- feeling pressured, irritable and easily upset

- feeling tense, agitated and 'on edge'

- difficulty concentrating

- difficulty staying on task and getting things done

- feeling overwhelmed and incompetent

- suffering from aches and pains

- feeling tired

- easily frustrated

- preoccupation with demands

- unproductive

- fragile and tearful, vulnerable

- appetite and sleep pattern changes.

Try some of the following to reduce stress in your life

- Eat healthily and get plenty of sleep to build up your body's stress tolerance.

- Decrease your intake of caffeine, alcohol and/or nicotine to prevent dependence on substances to cope with stress.

- Get regular exercise to vent frustration and release built-up tension.

- Take time each day to relax and unwind.

- Make time for leisure activities.

- Talk about how you are feeling with friends, family or a counsellor.

- Stand up for your rights, talk about what is bothering you and ask for changes to reduce your stress levels.

- Be assertive; do not be afraid to say no and to set limits upon how much you do.

- Set realistic goals and be kind to yourself, do not expect perfection.

- Look at the things that are causing you stress and make changes in the areas that you have control over. In the areas that you do not have control over, see if you can change the way you respond to them.

- Break tasks down into manageable steps and tackle them one at a time. Reward yourself as you achieve each step.

- Plan your time and use it wisely.

De-stressing your Thinking

Sometimes, the things that people say to themselves can contribute to their high levels of stress.

> **Think of a recent situation in which you felt stressed. What did you tell yourself?**

By changing the way you think when you are stressed, you can change the way you feel and cope with the situation. Try telling yourself some of these things next time you are feeling stressed:

- I can cope with this.
- I've done this before.
- What is the worst that could happen and could I cope with that?
- What do I want to achieve from this?
- I am going to beat this.
- There is no need to panic, I will get there.
- I will stay on top of this if I stay focused on my goal.
- I can only do the best I can and that's OK.
- I will do one thing at a time.
- No matter how stressed I feel, I always have options.
- I can choose to control this and to change this.
- If I cannot change the situation, I can change the way I respond to it.
- I have rights, I am important, I am doing well.
- I do not have to be perfect.
- Any mistakes I make are opportunities for learning.
- I will treat myself kindly and not with criticism or blame.
- Everything I cope with makes me a stronger person.
- I am in control of my life.

Things that Cause me Stress...

Write below a list of all the things in your life that cause you stress.

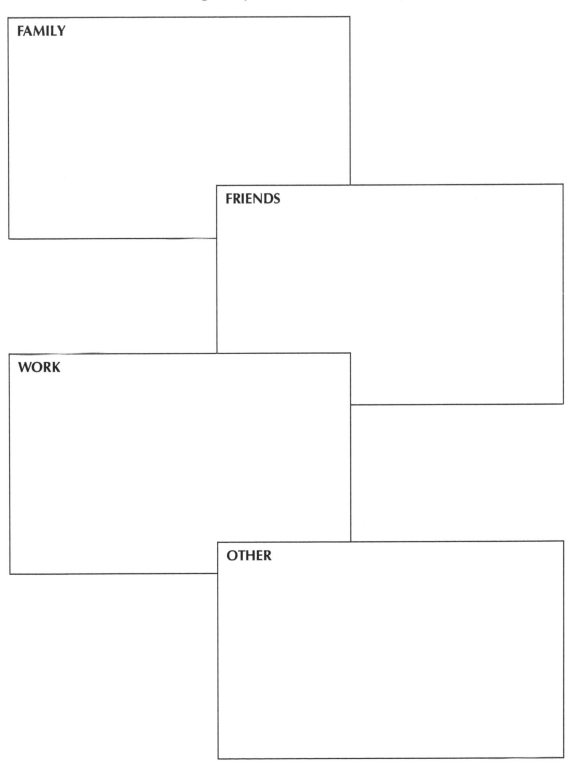

FAMILY

FRIENDS

WORK

OTHER

Balance

One important way to reduce stress is to make sure you have balance in your life, with generous amounts of work, rest, and play.

How much of your normal week do you spend on:

- **relaxation**

- **socialising**

- **recreation (hobbies)**

- **physical (sport/exercise)**

- **work/school**

- **spiritual/emotional fulfilment?**

Colour-code the above categories and then divide this pie chart into sections, showing how much time you spend on each category in a normal week.

What categories do you need to spend more time on?

How could you add this to your lifestyle?

Relaxation and Balance

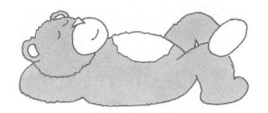

List below the activities you do to relax and how often you do them.

Relaxing/fun activities	How often do you do this?

What else could you do to relax, replenish, and have fun?

Pick some activities you could do daily, weekly and monthly to incorporate relaxation and fun in to your regular lifestyle:

Daily	Weekly	Monthly

8.3 Decision-making and time management

For clients to maintain treatment gains and to be able to cope with the challenges of life, they need to be aware of their needs and to be able to make good decisions. This section aims to help clients to be more aware of their needs and to consider their direction when making decisions.

Decisions

This sheet helps clients to weigh up the advantages and disadvantages of deciding to change. It is especially useful where the decision is whether to continue as they are or to risk making changes. This can be of use for a situation such as drug or alcohol abuse, where the client is trying to decide whether to continue using the substance as a coping mechanism or risk trying another strategy. It could also be used to help the client to decide whether to change jobs, let go of relationships, acquire a new possession, be honest with their family, let go of a strong belief system, etc. Decision-making is important in stress management and time management because it will help people to prioritise the pressures in their life and to think through the consequences of their decisions before they act.

Healthy and Unhealthy Situations

This sheet helps the client to identify situations that are healthy and unhealthy for them. Unhealthy situations are defined as those that prevent or threaten their goals for the future. Being aware of these situations early is imperative in preventing the negative consequences that they could cause. This can lead to careful planning and decision-making to increase the client's feeling of success and control over their life.

Time Management

This sheet asks the client to think about all the different aspects of their life that take up their time and to realistically examine how much time they need to allocate to each section of their life, the areas that could be cut down, and the areas that need more time. It also provides some tips for staying on task and for completing goals.

This sheet is aimed at clients who may be trying to juggle work, study, family, friends and more in their lives.

Weekly Planner

This is a blank timetable to help clients to plan their time to ensure that they balance their lifestyle and achieve their goals through healthy time management. This is most useful for setting up routines and for placing structure in the client's life.

'To Do' List

This list helps clients to keep track of their responsibilities by writing lists and breaking bigger tasks down into smaller steps. It encourages the client to plan for the day, the week and the month, to help them to remain on task. This increases their sense of control and mastery over their own life.

Decisions

What is it that I want to change?

_____

_____

Advantages	Disadvantages

Overall, is it better for you to change or to stay the same?

_____

_____

How can you do this?

_____

_____

Healthy and Unhealthy Situations

What are the most important things to you at present and for the future?

What situations/people/behaviours etc. could threaten these things?

What situations/people/behaviours etc. could help you to work towards these goals?

Time Management

Record on the table below all the different areas of your life that take up your time, e.g. family, friends, work, relaxation. Then think about how much of your time each area takes up and how much time you need to devote to that area of your life.

Area of your life	Time you currently spend	Time you need to spend

Time management tips

- Think about what changes you will need to make in order to devote more or less time to some of the areas of your life.

- To achieve bigger goals that you tend to put off, break them down into manageable steps and tackle them one at a time.

- Make lists of the things that you need to do and tick them off as you do them. Use planners, timetables and schedules.

- Reward yourself for any progress you make towards a goal.

- Balance work, rest and play to keep your mind fresh and your stress levels down.

Weekly Planner

Time	Monday	Tuesday	Wednesday	Thursday	Friday	Saturday	Sunday

'To Do' List

Tasks for the day								

Tasks for the week								

Tasks for the month								

8.4 Having direction

For the client to stay focused on their future goals and to stay on the track they have set themselves in therapy, it is important that they reflect upon the reasons for these goals and the benefits they are likely to receive by staying on task, and prepare for possible difficulties they may encounter. This section helps the therapist to explore these topics with the client in order to prepare them for termination of therapy and to help them to maintain treatment gains and develop further throughout their life.

What Really Matters to Me...

This is a sentence-completion task for clients to reflect upon what is important to them in their life and why. It asks them to think about the people who matter the most to them and what they personally have to teach others. It also focuses on what they need to do for themselves and why this is beneficial for them. These questions are very reflective and provide many opportunities for discussion and exploration by the client and the therapist.

My Direction for the Future

This sheet guides clients to reflect upon their long-term goals and to prepare for any possible pitfalls they may encounter that could hinder their progress. It aims to help the client to stay motivated to work towards their goals by reminding them of their reasons for setting them initially and by equipping them to deal with any possible pitfalls they may face. This should help to maintain the client's confidence as they work towards their goals and keep them on the course that they have set themselves.

Motivation

This sheet explores the concept of motivation by looking at the things that motivate clients and why, the things that drain their motivation and why, and what they can do to stay motivated to achieve their goals. This might lead to positive discussion about proactive strategies that the client can utilise in order to increase and maintain their motivation when confronting inevitable challenges in the future.

What Really Matters to Me...

The most important thing for me right now is _____

_____

What I want for my future _____

_____

The kind of person I want to become is _____

_____

The people I value the most are _____

_____

...because _____

_____

What I can teach others is _____

_____

The things I need to do for myself are _____

_____

These things are worth doing because _____

_____

My Direction for the Future

Where do you see yourself in five years' time?

Why is this important to you?

What steps do you need to take to get there?

What pitfalls might stop you from achieving these goals?

How can you plan to manage or avoid those pitfalls?

Motivation

What helps you to feel motivated? Why?

What drains your motivation? Why?

What happens when you are motivated?

What happens when you are unmotivated?

What can you do to prevent your motivation from being drained?

8.5 Preventing relapse

Developing a client's insight into their issues and equipping them with skills and strategies to reduce their discomfort is empowering for the client and immensely satisfying for the therapist. However, in order for their treatment gains to be maintained, clients need to be prepared for future trouble-spots they may encounter. This section aims to arm the client with skills to increase their self-awareness and to prepare specific responses to potentially difficult situations they may face after ending therapy.

Knowing your Weaknesses

This sheet asks the client to think about the things that make them most likely to engage in a target behaviour that has been reduced during therapy. For instance, a client who has been working on reducing angry outbursts might identify that alcohol increases the risk of this behaviour occurring. Similarly, this sheet could be used for clients who have increased a target behaviour through therapy, such as assertiveness. For these clients, the sheet could help them to explore the things that weaken their ability to perform the target behaviour (for example, conflict might weaken their resolve to voice their opinion assertively). By exploring these weaknesses, the client can plan how to manage them and stay in control. This helps them to stay on track and to prevent discouragement and disappointment.

Planning Ahead

In this exercise, the client is asked to think about three things they would like to keep working on in their life. They are prompted to look for obstacles that might prevent them from achieving their goals and what they could do to manage these. Finally, they are encouraged to plan how they will keep working on their goals. It is helpful for clients to think about their future goal achievement and personal development.

Reflection

This sheet provides an opportunity for very general reflection upon the client's learning experiences. It asks them what they have learned about themselves, what they need to focus on, and what they need to do to continue developing as a person. This sheet is deliberately vague so that it can be applied by the therapist to any setting or therapeutic question.

Therapy

This exercise aims to help clients to reflect upon their experience of therapy. It provides an opportunity to review their learning in therapy, what was most difficult for them in therapy, what they will continue to work on, and what was positive about the experience. This gives the therapist valuable feedback about the content and process of therapy, and helps to summarise the goals and outcomes of therapy for the client before termination.

Support

This sheet encourages clients to think about the people in their life who can support them in different ways. It asks them to think about the amount of support they receive from the important people in their life. It does this by asking clients to place the names of those who give them large amounts of support in the large hearts and those who give them limited support in the smaller hearts. The aim of this exercise is for the client to acknowledge the levels of support available to them and to make appropriate choices regarding whom they seek out for which kind and amount of support.

Dinner Party

This sheet asks clients to draw, using a symbol, all of the most important people in their life around a dinner table. This exercise aims to highlight the most important people in the client's life. The symbols that the client uses to describe each person can be informative, as can the seating of the guests respective to each other and the client. This task can elicit valuable information about the client's social support, family, and the relationships with and between the significant people in their life.

Warnings

This sheet asks the client to identify the signs that they may be slipping back into old patterns and might need to seek support from family and friends, or even return to therapy. The aim of this exercise is to increase the client's awareness of their behaviour and symptoms in order for them to act quickly and prevent relapse.

Warning, Warning, Warning!

This sheet asks the client to think of their warning signs that could indicate that they could be relapsing. It then asks them to generate some strategies to deal with each warning sign. This could be stuck up on a wall in a visible location to train the client to be vigilant to their warning signs so as to prevent or manage relapse.

Knowing your Weaknesses

Think of something that **you do** that you want to **reduce**

Why?

What are the things that make you most likely to do this behaviour?

How can you stop them from impacting on you?

Think of something that you **want to do more often**

Why?

What are the things that stop you from doing this?

How can you prevent them from stopping you?

Planning Ahead

What are three things you would like to continue working on in your life?

1. _____

2. _____

3. _____

Why are these things important to you?

What could stop you from working on these goals?

What steps could you take to ensure that you keep working on these goals?

1. _____

2. _____

3. _____

4. _____

5. _____

Reflection

What have you learned about yourself?

What do you need to focus on?

How can you continue to develop as a person?

Therapy

What was therapy like for you?

_____

_____

_____

What were the hardest things about therapy for you?

_____

_____

_____

What did you learn about yourself?

_____

_____

_____

What will you continue to work on after therapy? How will you do this?

_____

_____

_____

What were the most positive things about therapy?

_____

_____

_____

Support

Who do you have to support you in different ways in your life? Write their names into the hearts below. The different sized hearts represent different amounts of support.

Dinner Party

Think about the most important people in your life. Who would you invite to a dinner party in your honour?

Use a symbol to describe each person and draw them around the dinner table. Think about how you would place each guest, and don't forget to put yourself in!

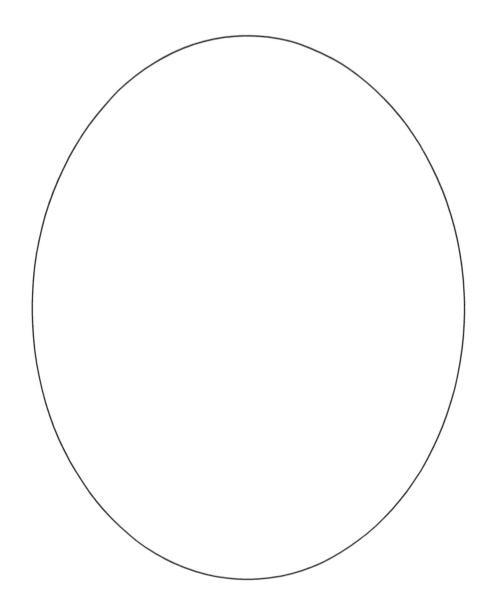

Warnings

How will you know when you might be slipping back into old patterns?

What signs will you notice in your body, thoughts and behaviour?

Will others be able to tell? How?

What do you need to do if you notice any of these warning signs?

Who can you go to for support if you need it?

Warning, Warning, Warning!

My warning signs	What I can do to manage this